HEARTBURN, BROKEN BONES, AND THE FALSE CLAIMS ACT

NATHAN V. TAKEDA PHARMACEUTICALS - WHY YOU SHOULD CARE ABOUT THE CASE YOU NEVER HEARD

NOAH NATHAN, MBA

CONTENTS

This book is dedicated to my sons Josh and Ben. I am so proud of both of them in how they have grown into young adults and continue to amaze me to this day. Although they were not directly involved with the case they were hugely affected by it. Their mother and I were obviously distracted due to the amount of time and attention we had to put into trying to do the right thing. They lost out on our time both physically and mentally and for that I am deeply sorry.

They have been brought up knowing how important it is to do the right thing and I hope that by reading this book they will know that we tried to teach by example.

I love you both!

PREFACE

The United States pharmaceutical market is the most important in the world, accounting for over 45 percent of global pharmaceutical sales, according to statista.com[1]. The United States, in 2016, spent $450 billion on medicine with 74 percent of the total cost for name brand products. It is easy to see why pharmaceutical companies would be tempted to break the rules.

This book is over nine years in the making, with a lot of peaks and valleys along the way. I have endeavored to write this book in order to tell my story of being a pharmaceutical whistleblower because the legal system prevented safeguarding the American public from potential health risks. My case was so compelling that it went all the way up to the United States Supreme Court but ultimately ended when the Court declined to intervene in my appeal. In writing this book, I have two important goals: (1) to make the public aware of a potential health risk that could affect thousands of Americans, and (2) to advocate for an amendment to the False Claims Act to enable future success in whistleblower suits. An amendment to the False Claims Act could remedy a disagreement of legal interpretations by different federal courts. This disagreement is hampering cases attempting to stop fraud against the government and to protect the public. Federal law should be the same throughout the country, but we have a problem.

To make you aware, I will be providing legal documents, court documents, government documents, articles from respected medical journals, facts from numerous sources, and some public information from Takeda Pharmaceuticals, the international corporation against which I brought suit. Throughout the book, I will strive to present the story in a way that will enable you to see the whole picture and take action to support laws that will protect the public.

My story is a David and Goliath tale wherein four people were trying to take on a multi-billion dollar corporation to do the right thing. In the process, we learned the hard way about how differing legal opinions affecting fraud cases are dividing the country.

This book is a call for action to clarify a portion of the False Claims Act (FCA). The American system of government provides a legislative branch that creates the laws, and a judicial branch that interprets the laws. President Abraham Lincoln signed the FCA into law during the Civil War to stop fraud against the government. This book will show how United States Courts are divided on the interpretation of a particularity issue in the Federal Rule of Civil Procedure 9(b) in the FCA. It can sound overwhelming, but Rule 9(b) creates the standard for the level of proof needed in fraud cases. The concern is that federal courts have differing interpretations of what meets that standard. The standards range from having knowledge and information about a fraud scheme on one end, up to possessing documents of the actual fraud on the other.

This amendment would not be the first time the FCA has been modified. The FCA has been updated multiple times since 1863. As recently as 2009, Congress did not agree with a Supreme Court's decision and passed the Fraud Enforcement and

Recovery Act (FERA) amendment to clarify the FCA. After reading my story, I hope you will be motivated to reach out to your elected officials and have them clarify the FCA so the courts can interpret it how President Lincoln intended, by stopping fraud against the government.

"I am a firm believer in the people. If given the truth, they can be depended upon to meet any national crisis. The great point is to bring them the real facts." Abraham Lincoln.

My case concerned how Takeda Pharmaceuticals instructed their sales representatives to promote dexlansoprazole. Dexlansoprazole is a proton pump inhibitor (PPI) sold under the brand name of Dexilant (it was initially called Kapidex, but due to some confusion at the pharmacy the name was changed. Throughout the book the drug will be referred to as both, but know they are the same). If you do a web search for "Nathan v. Takeda" you will find hundreds of hits and note how many times the decision in my case has been cited in other lawsuits (192 cites as of August 2018). Attorneys write most of the articles, and since the Supreme Court of the United States sent the case to the Solicitor General (SG) of the United States for his feedback, which is a rare occurrence, it got noticed. The U.S. Supreme Court receives an average of 7,000 cases annually, of which they will hear 70 and rule on another 50 without a hearing. They will only send 20 to the SG, as they did in my case. When the justices send a case to the SG's office, it is because there is a question about a significant legal issue and they want the executive branch's opinion.

When Kapidex launched in 2009, the sales data, as compiled by Takeda, did not specify the dosage at which it was prescribed. The sales for the 30mg and 60mg doses were grouped as a total sales number, which was a big issue since I couldn't prove what was written based on the reports. Eventually the company did provide dosage levels in its sales data, however, since it was during the case, we were not permitted to present the data as it became available. In my legal documents, I provided the knowledge and information about the fraud scheme along with statistical data to show the likelihood that the 60mg dose was written, where the 30mg dose was indicated. I explained that based on the fact that only the 60mg dose was promoted and sampled to doctors as a significant factor, but the court disregarded that argument. There is a process of gathering information leading up to a trial, and if allowed to continue with the process beyond the point at which my case was dismissed, the truth would have come out. In this book, I will establish my statistical information to be accurate and prove my case in the court of public opinion.

The case was significant to the legal community, but the medical community never heard about it, and thus, doctors were unaware of the risks to their patients. A study released in 2018 by *The Journal of Clinical Endocrinology & Metabolism* titled, "Fractures Tied to Increased Risk of Death for up to 10 Years"[2], spotlights the importance of the information in this book. The study shows that people over the age of 50 have an increase in mortality risk of up to 25 percent, after breaking a bone. There have been many studies regarding Proton Pump Inhibitors (PPIs) and bone fractures; enough of a concern that in May 2010 the Federal Drug Administration (FDA) required all PPIs to include a warning in their product labels about an increased risk of fractures of the hip, wrist, and spine. The FDA was so concerned about Dexilant and bone fractures that, to get the drug approved, Takeda was required to conduct a post-marketing study on bone fractures with Dexilant.[3] A post-marketing study means that after the product is available to the public, they will track a small percentage of patients taking the drug and compare them to patients not on the medication to determine if any negative response is the result of the specific medication. As of November 2018, the FDA website page concerning this study still shows, "No results posted."[4]

A study in the *Journal of the American Medical Association (JAMA)* from 2006 by Dr. Yu-Xiao Yang et al. titled, "Long-term

Proton Pump Inhibitor Therapy and Risk of Hip Fracture"[5] shows "Long-term PPI therapy, particularly at high doses, is associated with an increased risk of hip fracture." Another study in the *Journal of the American Medical Association (JAMA)* from 2009 by Dr. Carmen A. Brauer et al. titled, "Incidence and Mortality of Hip Fractures in the United States"[6] shows "about 30% of people with a hip fracture will die in the following year."

What this book will bring to light, is that without knowing about the PPI and bone fracture issue, the possibility that if a patient fell and broke a bone, they would not connect the medication's effect to their bones with the resulting injury. It is possible that a patient would not have broken a bone from the fall had they not been on such a high dose.

The main concern in recounting my story is that I fear the double dosing of Dexilant will be exposed as the reason for thousands of people to have broken bones including the hip, wrist, and spine as warned by the FDA. No results have been posted by the FDA, which is curious, given that the required deadline was years ago. Since the data hasn't been presented, I will be seeking independent data from the public by posting to my website: www.appleQD.com.

When Takeda was working on getting Dexilant approved by the FDA, they requested that 90mg be approved for erosive esophagitis and 60mg doses approved for maintaining healed erosive esophagitis and for GERD. The FDA rejected the 90mg dose but approved 60mg for erosive esophagitis and 30mg doses for maintaining healed erosive esophagitis and for GERD.[7] Takeda wanted 60mg to be indicated for the main reason PPI's are prescribed, GERD (heartburn). Even though the FDA refused to give the indication, Takeda instructed their sales representatives to encourage prescribing the 60mg treatment for GERD, where the FDA had approved only 30mg. GERD stands for GastroEsophageal Reflux Disease, better known as heartburn. I provided sworn statements to the court from several board-certified gastroenterologists, including a past-president of the American Medical Association, stating they were not aware that a 30mg dose of Dexilant existed until we reached out to them regarding the case.

Dexilant was replacing the heartburn drug Prevacid, a 3 billion dollars a year product for Takeda. As acknowledged by the President and CEO of Takeda Pharmaceuticals North America in a letter dated November 19, 2009, Mr. Shinji Honda stated, "Kapidex is building on Takeda's established presence in the PPI market. For more than a year, Takeda has been refocusing promotion, sales and sampling efforts to Kapidex."

A July 11, 2016, Takeda press release stated that over 28 million Dexilant prescriptions had been filled. In the years following that date, it is reasonable to assume that millions more have also been filled. According to Drugs.com, in 2014 there were 1.4 million Dexilant prescriptions filled in the three-month period of January - March, roughly 466,000 patients per month.[8] If you have experienced a broken bone of the hip, wrist, or spine from being on Dexilant 60mg (without ever trying the 30mg dose), I am deeply sorry that this information has not previously come to light. I tried to make these risks known, and as a failed whistleblower I have lost my career and my savings trying to do the right thing.

Why should you care about my story? Because as a whistleblower, I knew of a public safety risk that was being hidden and tried to do the right thing. A flawed legal system prevented my case from succeeding. Whistleblowers like me come forward when the general public is unaware that a safety issue exists, but please know that we are putting our careers on the line to bring these risks to light. There is a good chance that until hearing my story, you weren't aware of the health warning for Dexilant patients taking double the approved dose. Nor did you know that the federal courts in our country are split on how to interpret national law in fraud cases like mine.

During their defense, Takeda deflected any responsibility for double-dosing of Dexilant away from themselves and placed it on the physicians. Even though the physicians were not aware that a 30mg dose existed, Takeda claimed that they could have read the Dexilant package insert before prescribing.

In Takeda's Dexilant Sales Strategy Guide, they state that, "research and market history has shown a willingness by doctors to prescribe the highest marketed dose quickly after launch. Well over 90% of Prevacid and Nexium prescription volume is at the highest available dose per product." The Dexilant Sales Strategy Guide also reveals that, "there is a precedence in the class to only sample the highest available dose." The last statement has been shown to be inaccurate since the only PPI not to be sampled at more than one dose was Aciphex, which only comes in one strength. And finally, from the Dexilant Sales Strategy Guide, "we want patients to have the greatest opportunity for success especially since physicians may not know what they are treating initially (i.e. EE)." Erosive Esophagitis is only FDA approved at 60mg for 8 weeks, then the patient should be lowered to 30mg or taken off the medicine.

There is a relationship between pharmaceutical sales representatives and people in the medical field, where a trust is formed through information and the use of samples. The physicians were given 60mg samples, which was the only dose sampled, and told to give it to their GERD patients. The idea behind a sample is to make sure it works and is tolerated, so it is unrealistic to expect that a physician will provide a sample and then prescribe a different dose.

My name is Noah Nathan, and I am a whistleblower against Takeda Pharmaceuticals. In this book, I will take you through my rocky journey over 15 years working at Takeda including five years of my life as an active whistleblower working undercover with FBI and FDA agents, including wearing a wire during a three-day meeting in Arizona.

The primary desire to tell my story is to both, make the public aware of a potential health risk and advocate for an amendment to the False Claims Act. Additionally, I hope that this book will be of great interest and concern for the patients that have been taking Dexilant at the 60mg dose without ever trying the 30mg dose, the legal community, healthcare sales representatives, and health care providers to serve as a wake-up call to keep patient health as the main priority.

1

PROOF!

I was going to put this chapter towards the back of the book, but I feel it is essential for you to understand my frustrations early on. This information is from the timeframe during the case, but I was not able to introduce it into evidence. Even though Takeda knew the truth, they insisted my accusations were unprovable. Since it is too late to prove my case in a court of law, I will seek to prove it in the court of public opinion.

In an email to the sales force, Takeda openly admitted that 93% of Dexilant prescriptions were for the 60mg dose. Since, at that time, we didn't get the data broken down by dosage strength, I couldn't show that any prescriptions in my territory were written specifically for 60mg. Thus, it didn't pass the Rule 9(b) particularity standard of the 4th Federal Circuit Court needed to proceed.

My case was only interested in prescriptions that the government had to pay for. If private insurance companies want to be upset with this knowledge, it is their prerogative. To keep the math easy, I am only going to discuss Medicare Part D, but prescriptions reimbursed by Medicaid and Tricare would also fall under the lawsuit.

After the case became public and Takeda was aware of my involvement, they eventually took me off selling Dexilant and moved me to another medication. Because of this move, I don't have the sales numbers through when the Supreme Court declined to intervene in 2014, but I have enough information to prove my points. The following is 6 months of my sales data spanning October 2011 through March 2012:

Dexilant 60mg prescriptions 7,591

Dexilant 30mg prescriptions 302

In my territory, which was only 1 of 500, there were a total of 7,893 Dexilant prescriptions in the 6 months ending March 2012, 96% were for the 60mg dose.

The data I just provided was 6-month sales numbers ending in March 2012 for all Dexilant prescriptions in my territory. I am writing this book years later and don't have access to all of the data so I will have to jump around a little, but keep in mind, the longer the drug has been on the market, the more it is growing in use. A July 11, 2016, Takeda press release stated that over 28 million Dexilant prescriptions had been filled. In the years following that date, it is reasonable to assume that millions more have also been filled.

For the month of April 2011, there were 64 Medicare Part D prescriptions filled in my territory. At that time the data wasn't broken down by strength, but of the 64 only 27 were written by gastroenterologists and 0 were written by otolaryngologists - Ear Nose and Throat (ENTs) physicians. I mention gastroenterologists and otolaryngologists because they would be the only physicians that would have an indicated reason to prescribe Dexilant at the 60mg dose. The 60mg strength is ONLY indicated for erosive esophagitis and limited to eight weeks. In order to diagnose erosive esophagitis, a visual examination is required by inserting a camera scope into the patient's esophagus (throat) to see the damage. Of the physicians we called on, working for

Takeda, those were the only two specialties that would use a camera scope in their diagnosis.

So, of the 64 Medicare Part D prescriptions that were written, 27 could have been written for a proper indication, since they were prescribed by a gastroenterologist, leaving 37 prescriptions for the month that potentially were not prescribed for a proper FDA indication. Once the information was available, in every instance that the data was broken down by the 30mg and 60mg dose, it was always above 90% in favor of the 60mg strength. The fact that Takeda would claim that it is not "plausible" even after the information was known, I feel should be illegal.

According to an article by Dr. Amnon Sonnenberg in the *Yale Journal of Biology and Medicine*, "Clinical Epidemiology and Natural History of Gastroesophageal Reflux Disease"[1], looking at the patients "with GERD symptoms, about 20 percent are found to have erosive esophagitis, while ulcers or strictures are found in less than 5 percent of all patients with erosive esophagitis." What this information means, is that since only 20 percent of GERD patients have erosive esophagitis, the Dexilant 60mg sales data should be in that same 20 percent range, leaving Dexilant 30mg sales data at around 80 percent. The fact that 60mg sales are over 90 percent shows that it is due to the promotion and sampling of only that 60mg dose.

Looking at more information, this from the week ending January 18, 2013, shows the 10 weeks and the Fiscal Year To Date (FYTD: 4/1/12 through 1/18/13) as:

Dexilant 30mg 121 - 536

Dexilant 60mg 3,242 - 13,286

The percentages for 60mg are 96.4% for the 10 weeks and 96.1% for the FYTD.

In my Complaint, I mentioned 16 primary care physicians that had 98 Dexilant prescriptions filled by Medicare Part D. Takeda stated that I could not prove that those prescriptions were filled at the 60mg dose and that they must have been filled at the 30mg dose, which is what a primary care physician would write. The following are the physicians from my case, but this time I can show their prescribing habits. I will provide their information from January 2012 through December 2012 for both Dexilant 60mg and 30mg prescriptions, and I have Medicare Part D information for two of them. I feel that a rational, honest person will conclude that the prescriptions I showed in my original filing were for the 60mg dose.

The following are paragraphs from my Complaint with updated prescribing data included. Although my complaint named the specific physicians, I have blocked their names and will represent them as letters. I feel it is unfair to single them out since hypothetically, over 90 percent of Dexilant prescribing physicians throughout the country were also writing the 60mg dose. Knowing who they are is not a significant issue anymore, but the fact that I have the data to update their information is. Dexilant was initially named Kapidex, but due to confusion at the pharmacy level, the name was changed.

285. Relator conducted an analysis of a small amount of data from his territory (which is only 1 of 500 Takeda sales territories in the United States), for a limited time period (6 months) relating to one type of doctor (primary care physicians). From this data, Mr. Nathan identified 16 primary care physicians who received 60 mg samples at Takeda's direction, that each of these doctors prescribed Kapidex during the relevant period, and that these prescriptions resulted in 98 claims for Medicare reimbursement.

286. Dr. A wrote 33 prescriptions that were submitted to Medicare for reimbursement during this 6-month period, including 2 prescriptions for Kapidex in July 2010, 3 prescriptions in August 2010, 3 prescriptions in September of 2010, 4

prescriptions in October 2010, 7 prescriptions in December 2010, and 14 prescriptions in January 2011. Dr. A received 60 mg samples of Kapidex on July 14, 20, and 21, 2010, August 16, 2010, September 7, 10, 16, 17, and 29, 2010, October 4, and 26, 2010, November 11, and 15, 2010, December 17, 2010 and January 5, 14 and 20, 2011.

For January 2012 through December 2012 Dr. A wrote 1 Dexilant 30mg prescription and 180 Dexilant 60mg prescriptions.

287. Dr. B wrote 1 prescription that was submitted to Medicare for reimbursement during this 6-month period, writing 1 prescription in January 2011. Dr. B received 60 mg samples of Kapidex on May 12, 2010, August 23, 2010, September 16, and 30, 2010, October 11, 19, and 26, 2010, November 5, and 30, 2010, December 9, and 16, 2010, and January 6, 17, and 31, 2010.

For January 2012 through December 2012 Dr. B wrote 0 Dexilant 30mg prescriptions and 51 Dexilant 60mg prescriptions.

288. Dr. C wrote 2 prescriptions that were submitted to Medicare for reimbursement during this 6-month period, including 1 prescription for Kapidex in July 2010 and 1 in January 2011. Dr. C received 60 mg samples of Kapidex on April 8, 2010, May 27, 2010, July 9 and 19, 2010, September 2, 28 and 30, 2010, October 13 and 25, 2010, and January 17, 2011.

For January 2012 through December 2012 Dr. C wrote 0 Dexilant 30mg prescriptions and 45 Dexilant 60mg prescriptions.

289. Dr. D wrote 5 prescriptions that were submitted to Medicare for reimbursement during this 6-month period, including 2 prescriptions for Kapidex in October 2010, 1 in December 2010, and 2 in January 2011. Dr. D received 60 mg samples of Kapidex

on August 16, 2010, September 17 and 20, 2010, October 26 and 27, 2010, November 5, 2010, December 9, 2010, and February 7, 2011.

For January 2012 through December 2012 Dr. D wrote 0 Dexilant 30mg prescriptions and 9 Dexilant 60mg prescriptions.

290. Dr. E wrote 4 prescriptions that were submitted to Medicare for reimbursement during this 6-month period, including 1 prescription for Kapidex in July 2010, 1 in August 2010, 1 in September 2010, and 1 in January 2011. Dr. E received 60 mg samples of Kapidex on April 8, 2010, May 6 and 27, 2010, June 3 and 10, 2010, July 9 and 19, 2010, August 12, 2010, September 2, 9, 23, and 28, 2010, October 13, 21, and 28, 2010, November 4 and 23, 2010, December 2 and 16, 2010, and January 4, 2010.

For January 2012 through December 2012 Dr. E wrote 0 Dexilant 30mg prescriptions and 34 Dexilant 60mg prescriptions.

291. Dr. F wrote 2 prescriptions that were submitted to Medicare for reimbursement during this 6-month period, including 1 prescription for Kapidex in September 2010 and 1 in October 2010. Dr. F received 60 mg samples of Kapidex on May 11 and 21, 2010, August 11 and 26, 2010, September 1,7 and 13, 2010, October 11, 19 and 26, 2010, November 5, 23 and 30, 2010, December 9, 2010, January 4, 7, 20 and 28, 2011.

For January 2012 through December 2012 Dr. F wrote 0 Dexilant 30mg prescriptions and 19 Dexilant 60mg prescriptions.

292. Dr. G wrote 9 prescriptions that were submitted to Medicare for reimbursement during this 6-month period, including 2 prescriptions for Kapidex in July 2010, 1 in August 2010, 1 in September 2010, 2 in October 2010, 1 in December 2010, and 2 in January 2011. Dr. G

received 60 mg samples of Kapidex on August 20 and 27, 2010, September 10, 15, 22, and 29, 2010, October 4 and 18, 2010, November 1, 10, and 29, 2010, January 5, 2011, and February 1, 2011.

For January 2012 through December 2012 Dr. G wrote 21 Dexilant 30mg prescriptions and 83 Dexilant 60mg prescriptions.

293. Dr. H wrote 3 prescriptions submitted to Medicare for reimbursement during this 6-month period, including 1 prescription for Kapidex in August 2010, 1 in September 2010, and 1 in December 2010. Dr. H received Kapidex 60 mg samples on the following dates: June 10, 2010, July 9, 2010, August 19, 2010, September 2, and 13, 2010, October 13, 2010, November 23, 2010, and December 16, 2010.

For January 2012 through December 2012 Dr. H wrote 0 Dexilant 30mg prescriptions and 48 Dexilant 60mg prescriptions.

294. Dr. I wrote 4 prescriptions submitted to Medicare for reimbursement during this 6-month period, including 1 prescription for Kapidex in August 2010, 1 in September 2010, and 2 in October 2010. Dr. I received Kapidex 60 mg samples on the following dates: May 18, 2010, July 9, and 22, 2010, September 10, 2010, October 22, and 29, 2010, and December 10, 2010.

For January 2012 through December 2012 Dr. I wrote 0 Dexilant 30mg prescriptions and 4 Dexilant 60mg prescriptions.

295. Dr. J wrote 2 prescriptions submitted to Medicare for reimbursement during this 6-month period, including 1 prescription for Kapidex in August 2010 and 1 in September 2010. Dr. J received Kapidex 60 mg samples on the following dates: August 26, 2010, and November 4, 2010.

For January 2012 through December 2012 Dr. J wrote 0 Dexilant 30mg prescriptions and 16 Dexilant 60mg prescriptions.

296. Dr. K wrote 4 prescriptions submitted to Medicare for reimbursement during this 6- month period, including 2 prescriptions for Kapidex in August 2010, 1 in October 2010, and 1 in December 2010. Dr. K received Kapidex 60 mg samples on the following dates: May 24, 2010, July 7, 2010, August 23, 2010, October 5, 20, and 25 2010, November 12, 2010, December 13, 2010, and January 20, 2011.

For January 2012 through December 2012 Dr. K wrote 0 Dexilant 30mg prescriptions and 62 Dexilant 60mg prescriptions.

297. Dr. L wrote 3 prescriptions submitted to Medicare for reimbursement during this 6-month period, including 2 prescriptions for Kapidex in July 2010, and 1 in August 2010. Dr. L received Kapidex 60 mg samples on the following dates: May 10, 2010, September 1, and 27, 2010.

For January 2012 through December 2012 Dr. L wrote 0 Dexilant 30mg prescriptions and 6 Dexilant 60mg prescriptions.

298. Dr. M wrote 5 prescriptions submitted to Medicare for reimbursement during this 6-month period, including 4 prescriptions for Kapidex in July 2010 and 1 in August 2010. Dr. M received Kapidex 60 mg samples on the following dates: May 10, 2010 and August 27, 2010.

For January 2012 through December 2012 Dr. M wrote 1 Dexilant 30mg prescriptions and 18 Dexilant 60mg prescriptions.

299. Dr. N wrote 8 prescriptions submitted to Medicare for reim-

bursement during this 6-month period, including 2 prescriptions for Kapidex in July 2010, 2 in August 2010, 1 in September 2010, 2 in December 2010 and 1 in January 2011. Dr. N received Kapidex 60 mg samples on the following dates: June 1, 2010, July 14, 2010, August 20, 2010, October 5, 2010, November 11, 2010, December 13, 2010, January 10, and 24, 2011.

From January 2012 through December 2012 Dr. N wrote 0 Dexilant 30mg prescriptions and 78 Dexilant 60mg prescriptions, and of those 78 60mg prescriptions 19 of them were reimbursed through Medicare Part D.

300. Dr. O wrote 8 prescriptions submitted to Medicare for reimbursement during this 6-month period, including 1 prescription for Kapidex in July 2010, 2 in December 2010 and 5 in January 2011. Dr. O received Kapidex 60 mg samples on the following dates: May 5, 2010, June 7, and 29 2010, July 7, and 22, 2010, August 11, and 27, 2010, September 13, 2010, October 8, 2010, November 1, 8, and 22, 2010, December 6, 8, 13, 14, and 20, 2010, January 3, 12, and 19, 2010.

From January 2012 through December 2012 Dr. O wrote 2 Dexilant 30mg prescriptions and 180 Dexilant 60mg prescriptions, and of those 182 prescriptions, 26 of them were reimbursed through Medicare Part D.

301. Dr. P wrote 5 prescriptions submitted to Medicare for reimbursement during this 6-month period, including 1 prescription for Kapidex in July 2010, 1 in August 2010, 1 in September 2010, and 2 in October 2010. Dr. P received Kapidex 60 mg samples on the following dates: May 11, 2010, September 24, 2010, and October 28, 2010.

For January 2012 through December 2012 Dr. P wrote 0 Dexilant 30mg prescriptions and 2 Dexilant 60mg prescriptions.

. . .

OF THE 16 PHYSICIANS, 12 of them had 0 Dexilant 30mg prescriptions for January 2012 through December 2012.

My complaint had sales data, but it couldn't be broken down by the strength of dose. For those same 16 physicians I just showed their prescribing habits, but this time I could show what dose they chose to prescribe for their patients in 2012. Since only the 60mg dose was sampled and promoted, it is highly unlikely that the physicians mentioned above would have written 30mg during the time period of my filing then stopped and began writing 60mg right after. It should be obvious that if they didn't prescribe any Dexilant 30mg in 2012, it was not their choice previously either.

Takeda's Supreme Court Brief in Opposition was filed on July 12, 2013, seven months after the data I just provided showing what the physicians prescribed. In their brief dated July 12, 2013 they stated:

"THE COMPLAINT also identifies sixteen primary care doctors who received Kapidex samples and wrote ninety-eight Kapidex prescriptions that led to claims being submitted for reimbursement to Medicare, and twenty- five doctors of unknown specialties who received samples and wrote Kapidex prescriptions that were presented to Medicare Part D. Petitioner provides the month and year in which each doctor received samples and wrote Kapidex prescriptions that were purportedly presented to a federal program. Notably absent from these allegations, though, is any information regarding the condition for which the prescriptions were written, the dose of the prescriptions submitted for reimbursement, or any false statement by Takeda that led to the prescriptions. No allegations at all are made regarding the patients who were treated—e.g., whether they showed symptoms of GERD or whether EE was diagnosed or suspected. Petitioner alleges that 93% of all Kapidex prescriptions are at the 60 mg dose and that primary care physicians do not "regularly" treat the condition for which a 60 mg dose is approved. But he does not offer any comparable statistic focused on Kapidex prescriptions written by primary care physicians generally, or the physicians specifically named in the Complaint." *1 (The original version is at the end of the chapter, to make it easier to read I edited out the legal cites.)*

IN TAKEDA'S Dexilant Sales Strategy Guide, they state that, "research and market history has shown a willingness by doctors to prescribe the highest marketed dose quickly after launch. Well over 90% of Prevacid and Nexium prescription volume is at the highest available dose per product." The Dexilant Sales Strategy Guide also reveals that, "there is a precedence in the class to only sample the highest available dose." The last statement has been shown to be inaccurate since the only PPI not to be sampled at more than one dose was Aciphex, which only comes in one strength. And finally, from the Dexilant Sales Strategy Guide, "we want patients to have the greatest opportunity for success especially since physicians may not know what they are treating initially (i.e. EE)."

SOME QUOTES to point out from Takeda's opposition brief above are:

"Notably absent from these allegations, though, is any information regarding the condition for which the prescriptions were written, the dose of the prescriptions submitted for reimbursement".

Due to the Health Insurance Portability and Accountability Act (HIPAA) regulations, pharmaceutical representatives would not have legal access to that information. As of 2012, seven months before their brief was written, they were aware of the doses that those physicians prescribed but maintained that the physicians must have written Dexilant at the 30mg dose.

"No allegations at all are made regarding the patients who were treated—e.g., whether they showed symptoms of GERD or whether EE was diagnosed or suspected."

Again, due to HIPAA regulations, not myself or any other pharmaceutical representative, would have legal access to that information.

"Petitioner alleges that 93% of all Kapidex prescriptions are at the 60 mg dose".

This is not something that I alleged, this is what was provided to me, as well as the entire sales force, via email from Takeda management and documented in the case. Also notable, after the fact, is that in my territory, Dexilant 60mg was written over 95% of the time.

It is important to point out that my case was lost at the "motion to dismiss" stage. I had enough information to show the issue and if I had been able to continue with the case most of the issues that they claim can't be proven, would have been.

One of Takeda's main defenses was that the price for Dexilant 30mg and 60mg were the same; thus Takeda was not making more profit by pushing the 60mg over the 30mg. Takeda brought this price issue up several times in their opposition brief trying to make a point that without the profit motive, I had no case. I tried to show that the reason Takeda wanted the 60mg is that it is more likely to have a positive response for the patient causing the patient to continue to refill their prescriptions. By refilling their prescriptions, Takeda will continue to increase its revenue from sales of the product. If the patient took the 30mg and it did not have a positive response, the patient may choose to switch to another product causing Takeda to lose revenue.

*1

"The Complaint also identifies sixteen primary care doctors who received Kapidex samples and wrote ninety-eight Kapidex prescriptions that led to claims being submitted for reimbursement to Medicare, and twenty- five doctors of unknown specialties who received samples and wrote Kapidex prescriptions that were presented to Medicare Part D. Id. at 104a–109a (¶¶ 284–301), 111a–116a (¶¶ 315–40). Petitioner provides the month and year in which each doctor received samples and wrote Kapidex prescriptions that were purportedly presented to a federal program. Id. at 105a–109a (¶¶ 286–301), 111a–116a (¶¶ 315–40). Notably absent from these allegations, though, is any information regarding the condition for which the prescriptions were written, the dose of the prescriptions submitted for reimbursement, or any false statement by Takeda that led to the prescriptions. No allegations at all are made regarding the patients who were treated—e.g., whether they showed symptoms of GERD or whether EE was diagnosed or suspected. Petitioner alleges that 93% of all Kapidex prescriptions are at the 60 mg dose (Id. at 67a (¶ 128)) and that primary care physicians do not "regularly" treat the condition for which a 60 mg dose is approved. Id. at 84a–85a (¶¶ 208–09). But he does not offer any comparable statistic focused on Kapidex prescriptions written by primary care physicians generally, or the physicians specifically named in the Complaint. "

$42 BILLION

The False Claims Act (FCA), also called "Lincoln's Law", was designed to have the reward as a significant part of the incentive for the whistleblower to come forward. The False Claims Act was signed into law during the Civil War by President Abraham Lincoln to stop contractors from committing fraud against the Union. I will get into more details of the FCA in a later chapter, but the numbers in this chapter should be an eye-opener and peak your interest in my story.

It is essential to keep in mind the growth of Dexilant over the years. A July 11, 2016, Takeda press release stated that over 28 million Dexilant prescriptions had been filled. In the years following that date, it is reasonable to assume that millions more have also been filled. According to Drugs.com[1], in 2014 there were 1.4 million Dexilant prescriptions filled in the three-month period of January - March, roughly 466,000 patients per month.

Since I would have the actual data if the case went forward and not have to look through old reports, I will use the big picture view to interpret the numbers. In February 2011, when Dexilant was still growing, in the Charlottesville, VA district, which consists of 3 of the 500 Takeda territories in the U.S., there were a total of 1,891 Dexilant prescriptions for the month. Of those 1,891 Dexilant prescriptions, 150 were for Medicare Part D, 5.33%. In March 2011, for the same district, the totals were 2,123 and 187 for Medicare Part D, 6.01%. Now, not every prescription reimbursed through Medicare Part D would have been an off-label prescription. An off-label prescription means the way the medication is written was not for an FDA approved use.

In determining what the penalty would be today, since it is just funny money anyway lets say 50% was off-label, where it is probably up around 80%. If we take only the 28 million prescriptions of Dexilant that were filled through 2016, from Takeda's own press release, and assume 5% were for Medicare Part D, that totals 5.6 million prescriptions. Since we are considering that only 50% are for off-label use, that is 2.8 million prescriptions which Takeda is responsible for.

In False Claim Act cases the damages are $5,000 to $10,000 for each infraction, and since it is a *qui tam* fraud case, it is treble damages (3 times). Taking 2.8 million infractions at $5,000 each, to use the low end to be generous, it totals $14 billion. And when we add the treble damages, it totals $42 BILLION!

The False Claims Act law establishes that the whistleblower is entitled to 15-30% of what the government takes in. If the government declines to intervene in the case, which happened in mine, the whistleblowers share increases to a minimum of 25% with a maximum of 30%. Again, keeping to the lowest factor, let's assume 25% of the government's recovery of $42 Billion, my share would have been $10.5 Billion. These are numbers through 2016, my case ended in 2014 with the U.S. Supreme Court declining to hear my appeal. At the time, we were estimating that the case would have been worth about $2 Billion. If we would had moved forward with the case and won, Takeda would have settled with the Department Of Justice for less than the $2 billion, and we would have received our portion from that. It would have been more than enough compensation and been a full-time job giving the money away to worthy causes.

THE PHARMACEUTICAL INDUSTRY

I began my career in pharmaceutical sales in 1998. In the 1990's and the early 2000's being a pharmaceutical sales representative was a highly sought after position with high pay and prestige. As sales representatives, we had the freedom of being on our own, driving from office to office without any immediate supervision or anyone to answer to. Usually, a manager would spend the day with you about once a month with a few conference calls mixed in, but mainly you were on your own with a company car and an expense account.

It is a common practice to bring lunch to physician offices to provide information about specific medications. Meals are one of the best ways to get access to the physicians as well as the other vital members of the office. Some offices have a different representative bringing lunch every day!

Aside from lunches, the primary way pharmaceutical sales representatives interact with physicians is when they are between patients. Most people reading this has been in a situation when you were in a doctor's office for an appointment, and they are running behind. You have to deal with the frustration of being there on time, they are now 30 minutes past your scheduled appointment, and in walks a happy go lucky pharmaceutical sales representative. In your mind, that representative is going to see your physician causing you to wait even longer which is really pissing you off! I have had patients come up and ask me to wait until they see their doctor before I go back and try and talk to him.

In reality, we usually only get 15 seconds to 1 minute with the physicians as they sign for the samples going from patient room to patient room. It is our job to come up with interesting open-ended questions to turn a 30-second visit into a 4 to a 5-minute conversation about how our medication can benefit their patients as well as make life easier for them and their office staff.

One important note I need to make is that to keep this book as easy to read as possible, I will use the term physician and doctor to refer to medical personnel who can write prescriptions. I want to make sure mid-level practitioners receive their due credit in their benefit to the healthcare system. Nurse Practitioners and Physician Assistants diagnose and care for their patients and prescribe medication as needed. For most appointments, there isn't any difference in the result you would get if you saw a mid-level or your doctor. Without mid-level practitioners, the health system would come to a slow crawl, and sick patients would not get treated in a timely fashion.

In the pharmaceutical industry, the products have defined life cycles; Launch, Growth, Maturity, and Decline. In the launch phase, which is considered the first year on the market, it is imperative to grow usage quickly and have physicians agree to prescribe for their patients. We need them to use the product so they can get the first-hand experience from their patients if it is working or not. If they get positive feedback from their patients, they will be more willing to use it on other patients thus growing the business. In a chronic medication, patients will be refilling the prescriptions monthly allowing for substantial growth as more patients begin the drug. At the same time, if it doesn't work or has adverse side effects, they will not use it and may never try it again.

Sampling is essential for new products, and are provided so physicians can get experience and patient feedback with limited patient financial risk in case the drug doesn't work. The main reason a launch is so important is that once a patient is on the medicine with success, they will typically stay on it and continue to get refills. Refills are the key to any chronic condition. Antibiotics are usually taken as a temporary problem, and the pharmaceutical company needs to make their money on the handful of pills necessary to treat the infection whereas a chronic condition could mean the patient remains on the medicine for years if not indefinitely.

Another critical factor of a good launch is in dealing with insurance companies. If the pharmaceutical company can show how strong the drug launch is going, and how well patients are doing on it, then the insurance company should put it on the preferred status of their formulary. If the drug had a bad launch with few patients, the insurance carrier might put it as a tier-3 with a higher co-pay, as a non-preferred status with an even higher co-pay, or possibly not covering it at all.

The growth phase is once the product has been on the market for a year and lasted until the increase in sales flattens out. During the growth phase, the company continues to invest in promotional efforts consisting of advertising, samples, and representative face time to increase sales. This phase will last for several years depending on the product and the company. If a company has several products in this phase, they might decide to give more effort to the one that is more profitable and/or reach out for a promotional partner.

The maturity phase is when the product has flattened out and has barely started to decline in sales. In this phase, the product is going well, and the number of promotional dollars spent will not be recouped in additional sales. Because of the low or negative return on investment, companies will reduce promotion until the next phase of the lifecycle, decline.

The final phase of the pharmaceutical product lifecycle is decline. At this stage, the company stops the promotional spending with the anticipation that sales will be consistent until the patent expiration and generics take over the product.

The majority of pharmaceutical sales occur through the physician writing a prescription and the patient filling it at a pharmacy. (An example of a transaction not through the pharmacy is when a product is given to a patient through an IV in the physician's office) This makes crediting sales data a little complicated since it isn't a direct sale model. There are third party companies who purchase the data from pharmacies and sell it to pharmaceutical companies to compensate the sales representatives appropriately as well as provide valuable information on what individual physicians prescribe. Knowing what the physician prescribes is extremely important in "pre-call planning" while determining how to influence their prescribing habits. The data is 2-3 months delayed since the third party needs to match the prescription up to the physician without forwarding any patient information, which would be against HIPAA.

Physicians can opt-out of having pharmaceutical companies know their prescribing habits, but most are not concerned with it. The fact that we know what they write is usually something that is not talked about; however, there are some that will comment on their prescribing habits. The frustrating thing is when you have a physician that is telling you they are writing but the data doesn't show it. I have had some physicians who would comment that they have been writing a lot of product X lately and ask if the information is showing it?

Pharmaceutical representatives can categorize physicians in several different groups. The main differentiators are if they are a primary care physician office or a specialty medical office, an office that prescribes a lot of branded medication compared to an office that uses mostly generics, an office that accepts certain insurances that your drugs are easily approved on, and if the office allows representatives access to the physicians. More and more physician offices are closing access to sales representatives. The lack of access is partially due to the increased demand for the offices to see more patients and they can't afford the time talking to sales representatives. With insurance reimbursement being reduced, this causes the physicians to see more patients just to break even. Some offices have banned sales representatives because they were becoming too aggressive, with some representatives even pushing their products right in front of patients. The new trend is to only allow sales representatives during lunch, with the representative providing a meal for the entire office.

Beginning in 2013, the Physician Payments Sunshine Act requires manufacturers of drugs and medical devices, that participate in U.S. federal health care programs, to track and report certain payments and items of value to the Centers for Medicare and Medicaid Services on an annual basis. The Sunshine Act began reporting on August 1, 2013, which spooked some physicians into no longer accepting lunches in their offices so they wouldn't be seen as taking gifts to prescribe certain medications. The leading physicians on the list are official product speakers that are paid by the pharmaceutical companies.

The website is https://openpaymentsdata.cms.gov/search/physicians/by-name-and-location.

The physician with an enormous amount that I know is an Endocrinologist that speaks for a lot of pharmaceutical companies. I won't mention his name, but he is an excellent speaker and a well-respected physician. According to the website, in 2015, he made $570,238 but minus expenses he was paid $428,285 for speaking fees.

Pharmaceutical representatives aren't allowed to ask or offer a *quid pro quo* for the physicians to write prescriptions, but there is a strong emphasis for a return on our investment (ROI). The main investments/expenses that are tracked include pharmaceutical samples and meals. Although there is no charge to the physician for samples, they do cost the company millions of dollars annually to produce in special packaging. The number of office visits by a sales representative is seen as an additional expenditure on investment since the company is paying the representatives salary and requires a certain number of office visits on a daily basis.

Pharmaceutical samples vary but are usually packaged in a 7-day container. The goal is that the physician will write a prescription and give a sample to the patient to make sure the product is tolerated before getting the prescription filled at the pharmacy. At times an excessive amount of samples are provided to the patient even without a prescription, meaning the company and the representative won't get any credit but makes the physician a great guy for giving away hundreds of dollars of free medication.

Depending on the medication and disease state, samples can play a different important role. With antibiotics, the typical number of pills indicated to resolve the infection could range from 1 to 20 for newer medications. The idea for sampling antibiotics is the quicker the patient starts them, the faster they will feel better. It also allows for the patient to initiate the antibiotic right in the physician's office without the need to rush to the pharmacy that day. The downside is when the provider gives a full course of therapy away, and no credit is given for the sales representative's effort. That is the main issue regarding samples when comparing acute, short duration, to chronic, longer duration, medical conditions. In chronic diseases, the primary benefit of a sample is to make sure the patient doesn't have an adverse reaction to the medicine. The timeframe to see results differs from disease state to disease state with chronic condition results noticed more by medical testing compared to how the patient is feeling. Since the physician doesn't want to waste their time as well as the patient's, they will schedule a follow-up visit a month later to evaluate the medication's benefits. With a 7-day sample, the patient will know if they tolerate the drug and can have the prescription filled to continue the therapy. However, some offices will give the entire month of samples and write the medicine at the follow-up visit.

The offices that receive a lot of samples and do not show up as writing prescriptions, get flagged, and the representative has to explain the situation to their superiors. In some cases these offices are in low-income areas where the patients can't afford the medication, maybe the offices just want to give them away to their patients since they didn't cost them anything, possibly the office staff uses them, and sometimes the third party tracking system just doesn't catch that the prescriptions were written and filled. Regardless of the reason, the representatives are responsible for the samples they give out.

When I began in pharmaceuticals, we could offer meals and snacks to physicians without needing to have them sign any documents. Actually, we could take physicians golfing, to baseball games, etc...... I had two doctors that golfed every Wednesday afternoon, and the representatives would sign up in advance on who would take them out. The good thing about that was the company would pay me to play at the nicer courses, and I would get 4 to 5 hours of face time to talk about the benefits of my medications. Things have changed, and representatives aren't even allowed to provide pens anymore so that the *quid pro quo* would not be questioned. When we give a meal or snack, everyone taking part must sign a sheet acknowledging the fact they are consuming a meal and certify that they are not a government employee. On our expense reports, this information is documented and tracked for company purposes as well as The Sunshine Act.

So we can't look for a *quid pro quo*, but we do need to be aware of our return on investment. This is a fine line, but it is business.

It is essential to keep in mind that healthcare is a business and the physician office needs to be profitable. Martha Rosenberg, from centerforhealthjournalism.org, wrote an article titled, "The changing role of the pharmaceutical representative."[1] She reported on a talk between Dr. Audiey Kao, Vice President of Ethics at the American Medical Association and Dr. Richard Pinckney, a professor at the University of Vermont College of Medicine, from a 2010 conference. Dr. Pinckney talked about the challenge of refusing patients medicinal requests calling it "Refusal skills." He said writing a prescription is easy but, "explaining to a patient why a highly advertised drug might not be appropriate only takes three minutes." Dr. Kao shared that, "Doctors have a hard time saying no if a drug is effective, even if it is expensive." In response, Dr. Pinckney agreed and revealed, "Doctors are "nervous" that rebuffed patients will go elsewhere."

Dr. John Abramson described his dilemma as a practicing physician in his book Overdo$ed America[2]. Dr. Abramson explains the predicament he was in with one of his patients demanding a prescription for Celebrex to cure his tennis elbow, solely based on a friend's recommendation. Dr. Abramson tried to help his patient by giving him some exercises along with an inexpensive NSAID, both of which have been proven to work for his issue. Unfortunately, the patient made it very clear that either he left with a prescription for Celebrex or he would find another physician who would. Against his better judgment, Dr. Abramson wrote the prescription.

Pharmaceutical representatives work from home and depending on their living situation, will keep their samples and other sales supplies in their home or at a temperature controlled storage shed location. Territories differ in size depending on their geography and are usually broken down to the number of target offices to be called on. In rural areas, the region could stretch 200 or more miles across compared to territories in Manhattan measured in blocks. Representatives would call on around 200 to 250 physicians in their territory with some being seen more than others. We used to keep notebooks, which eventually became computer notes when laptops started being used. The benefits of notes are so you could document what you talked about, and if the physicians brought up any objections, you could follow up with them on the next visit. If you have a sales partner, they can see what you talked about and can progress from there. It can be challenging to keep track of 200 to 250 physicians while you have so many different conversations every day. The company eventually took away our ability to take notes from our sales calls because when the company would get sued, the records would be part of the discovery process to show what the representatives discussed with the physicians, primarily if they spoke off-label.

Hollywood has made several attempts portraying pharmaceutical sales representatives, and most of them are pretty accurate to a point. If you want to see some funny characterizations from the representative's perspective, do an internet search for, "Charles Charles pharmaceutical."

Jake Gyllenhaal's role in "Love and Other Drugs" has some very realistic scenes. During his initial sales training, he lights a match and tries to get through his product information before it burns his fingers. As I mentioned earlier the usual time we get in front of a physician is 15 seconds to 1 minute, so it is important to be able to get out a quick sales call when we are in front of the provider. Our primary job is to turn the quick call into a valuable discussion. The better relationships you have with the physicians, the more time you can get, which is why when you change companies they want to know which offices you already have good relationships with to gain better access with their products.

An important overlooked part of pharmaceutical sales is being able to interact with the entire office. The physician writes the prescription, but it is a team effort at times to get it approved and into the hands of the patient. Jake Gyllenhaal's character was very good at this except for the scene where he was handing out Viagra samples to everyone since they need to be signed for by a physician as a controlled substance. Basically, think of any drug that you can't buy over the counter is a controlled substance.

"The Big Bang Theory" has Penny as a pharmaceutical sales representative and that is the usual stereotype, a beautiful young woman pushing medicine deemed not that important. Some representatives were cheerleaders in high school, and college and the majority of them are attractive, but they still need to know their information. That being said, at annual sales meetings, it can be hard to tell the difference between a pharmaceutical or modeling conference.

According to Medreps.com[3], "While the movies often portray pharma sales reps as beautiful women rolling a suitcase into doctors' offices, the image is a large misrepresentation. In fact, only 31 percent of pharma sales reps are women." Medreps provided some interesting data in their report titled "2017 Pharmaceutical Sales Salary Report". The report shows that in 2017 the average compensation for a pharmaceutical sales representative is $128,490 and $147,318 for a specialty pharmaceutical representative. (See the information at the end of the chapter for more details.) In my experience, it is very accurate with a lot of older representatives continuing to stay in the industry for the main reason that they can't make that kind of money elsewhere. Through the years of blockbuster medications going off-patent and massive layoffs, the representatives that survived have benefited financially.

Although it is illegal to terminate older employees based on their age, it is clear that companies can save a lot of money by hiring younger employees for half the cost. The main benefit seasoned representatives bring is their relationships with the physicians and their offices. Access is gold in the pharmaceutical world. If you can't inform the physicians about your products, there is a good chance they will not be prescribed or prescribed enough to meet your sales goals. Due to an increased workload, many offices have been limiting representative access, and there is no sign of that changing course.

Pharmaceutical companies are expanding to online media to try and educate the physicians about their products. There are email lists they can sign up for as well as specific parts of the product websites that are designed for physician use compared to patient use. There is usually no barrier to stop a patient from viewing the information intended for physicians, but they assume that either the patient will not understand the data or just be bored by it. Try it yourself, check out the website of a medicine you are taking and look for the HCP (Health Care Provider) or Physician link. Click on it and see how much you understand or if it makes you feel better about medicine that you are ingesting.

An interesting fact stated by Elisabeth Rosenthal in her book, "An American Sickness: How Healthcare Became Big Business and How You Can Take It Back,"[4] the United States is one of only two countries that allow certain forms of drug advertisement, the other being New Zealand.

Although they are not always followed, many regulations limit pharmaceutical companies on what they are allowed to say on their websites, in print, and verbally. Unfortunately, as shown by multiple pharmaceutical settlements with the government, representatives will speak off-label promoting their drugs to gain more prescriptions. There are rules but as I will get into they are not always followed.

When I mention, "off-label" I am referring to what is written and approved by the FDA in the product's package insert. Representatives are only allowed to talk about what is in the package insert. There may be additional studies and updated package inserts but only approved data and indications can be discussed with physicians. If off-label questions come up, there is a process to follow. Most of the time the representative would fill out a form, which the physician must sign stating that they brought up the question without being prompted, and someone from the home office will get back to them. Another option is to have a Doctor of Pharmacy (PharmD) employed by the company, contact the physician with the question and answer their unsolicited off-label question.

In the 1990's pharmaceutical consultants told the companies that they need more, "share of voice" in the physician offices to grow their market share. Pfizer and Merck had so many representatives in the field that you would see several representatives with the same medicines on any given day. This growth in sales representatives put a strain on physician offices having to be aware of representative access to the sample closet, to assure only one at a time, along with keeping the physicians on schedule. Pfizer's drug Lipitor was making over $10 Billion annually before it went generic and lost its patent. When these blockbuster drugs went generic, the pharmaceutical industry began to shrink, and massive layoffs ensued.

According to www.pharmaceuticalcommerce.com[5], there were around 102,000 pharmaceutical sales representatives in the U.S. during 2005 as a high and down to approximately 62,000 in 2013 as a low. In 2017 there were about 70,000 pharmaceutical sales representatives. Access to physicians has been declining and continued to do so. In 2009 access was around 80% that the sales representatives could see the physicians but it has been less than 50% in recent years.

To get an idea of who pharmaceutical representatives really are, Medreps.com conducted a survey in 2017 with 666 respondents: https://www.medreps.com/medical-sales-careers/pharmaceutical-sales-salary-report.

Medreps.com[6] showed that the average salary for pharmaceutical sales representatives is $128,489 and specialty pharmaceutical sales representatives earn $147,318. The data they compiled has the age breakdown as:

20-30: 9%

31-40: 28%

41-50: 41%

51-60: 20%

60+: 2%

The average salary based on age is:

20-30 years old: $98,049

31-40 years old: $131,358

41-50 years old: $144,868

51-60 years old: $143,674

60+ years old: $161,864

Years of experience in pharmaceutical sales is represented as:

<2 years: 8%

2-5 years: 16%

6-10 years: 13%

11-20 years: 45%

20+ years: 18%

The respondents were 61% male with an average salary of $144,025 and 39% female with an average salary of $126,681.

4
___

THE FOOD AND DRUG ADMINISTRATION

The United States Food and Drug Administration is a federal agency of the United States Department of Health and Human Services. The FDA is responsible for protecting the public health by assuring the safety, effectiveness, quality, and security of human and veterinary drugs, vaccines and medical devices.

The FDA regulates the manufacture and marketing of prescription medicines to protect the public's health and safety under the Food, Drug, and Cosmetic Act. Under the FDCA and implementing regulations, no new drug can be introduced into interstate commerce until the FDA has determined that it is "safe and effective" for its intended uses and approved its marketing and sale.

Companies seeking to market a new drug in the U.S. must submit a New Drug Application (NDA) to the FDA. According to the FDA[1], all new drugs sold in the U.S. since 1938 have gone through the approved NDA process. Data gathered during animal studies, and human clinical trials become part of the drug's NDA, which will be used by the FDA reviewer to reach the following key decisions:

• Whether the drug is safe and effective in its proposed use(s), and whether the benefits of the drug outweigh the risks.

• Whether the drug's proposed labeling (package insert) is appropriate, and what it should contain.

• Whether the methods used in manufacturing the drug and the controls used to maintain the drug's quality are adequate to preserve the drug's identity, strength, quality, and purity.

THE DOCUMENTATION REQUIRED in an NDA is supposed to tell the drug's whole story, including what happened during the clinical tests, what the ingredients of the drug are, the results of the animal studies, how the drug behaves in the body, and how it is manufactured, processed and packaged.

ONCE THE FDA approves a drug for a particular use, doctors may prescribe the drug for other uses, referred to as "off-label" uses. "Off-label" refers to the use of an approved drug for any purpose, or in any manner, other than the indications and dosages approved by the FDA and described in the drug's labeling. Off-label use includes treating beyond the indications and uses, treating the indicated condition at a different dose or frequency than specified in the label, or treating a different patient population (e.g., treating a child when the drug is only approved to treat adults). The FDA allows physicians to prescribe off-label in an effort to avoid interfering with their practice of medicine. However, physicians who practice off-label medicine are responsible for the outcomes. While physicians may prescribe off-label, companies are expressly prohibited from marketing or promoting drugs for off-label uses. To keep it simple, companies can only promote a drug for what is in the FDA approved package insert.

The main point of my case was that Takeda is promoting

Dexilant off-label by marketing the 60mg dose for GERD. The Dexilant package insert clearly states that 60mg is only indicated for erosive esophagitis for 8 weeks. The 30mg dose is indicated for maintaining healed erosive esophagitis and for GERD. In their New Drug Application, Takeda asked for 90mg to heal erosive esophagitis and 60mg for maintaining healed erosive esophagitis as well as for GERD. The FDA only approved the 60mg for healing erosive esophagitis and 30mg for maintaining healed erosive esophagitis and GERD. Takeda didn't promote and sample the 30mg dose until many years later, and that was in a limited role.

To limit confusion, I will add this clarifying information several times throughout the book. Dexilant was initially approved under the name Kapidex but was changed in 2010 to avoid confusion with a similar sounding medication. Kapidex was approved for the company TAP Pharmaceuticals that stood for Takeda Abbott Partnership Pharmaceuticals. TAP was split between Takeda and Abbott with Dexilant becoming part of Takeda Pharmaceuticals.

TAP Pharmaceuticals submitted its New Drug Application (NDA) for Kapidex in December 2007. In its NDA, TAP sought approval of 30, 60 and 90 mg dosages of Kapidex. In 2009, the FDA approved 60mg for healing erosive esophagitis for 8 weeks and 30mg for maintaining healed erosive esophagitis and 30mg for GERD.

There were several doctors at the FDA working on the NDA for Kapidex. Two leading FDA researchers for Kapidex were Dr. Keith B. St. Amand and Dr. Tamara Johnson. In Dr. St. Amand's summary, as noted on the FDA website concerning the Risk/Benefit Assessment[2]:

"SINCE THIS REVIEW evaluated only the efficacy of the product, it is difficult to provide a detailed risk/benefit assessment here. However, the reviewer is aware of several safety concerns that have arisen with this application (see Dr. Tamera Johnson's review of safety). Although dexlansoprazole is effective for all 3 indications being sought, the reviewer strongly believes that no convincing evidence of additional benefit over existing therapies has been demonstrated in the current application."

"Due to this lack of additional benefit along with the safety concerns that have been voiced in Dr. Johnson's review, the reviewer believes that the benefit/risk profile for dexlansoprazole is unfavorable at this time, and that future studies should be required to clarify the nature of the potential safety signal before any approval for marketing is granted."

Dr. Tamara Johnson's Risk/Benefit Assessment shows concern for both safety and "benefit over the 5 currently marketed PPI's":

"Dexlansoprazole belongs to the drug class of proton pump inhibitors (PPI); a class which now houses 5 marketed products (see section 2.2.) Throughout its Phase 3 development program, dexlansoprazole has demonstrated a greater benefit for the symptomatic GERD and the erosive esophagitis patient populations when compared to placebo and lansoprazole (Prevacid) 30mg. Although, as discussed in the efficacy review by Dr. St. Amand, dexlansoprazole provides no additional benefit over the 5 currently marketed PPI's, the benefit of dexlansoprazole outweighs the risk of adverse events. Safety concern about a potentially increased risk of ischemic cardiovascular adverse events among dexlansoprazole 30mg subjects was diminished due to previous cardiac medical history in the subjects and absence of similarly increased risk among dexlansoprazole 60mg and 90mg treatment groups. Labeling recommendations have been advised to address this potential concern. This reviewer, however, remains with concern for fracture/injury-related adverse events, which occurred at greater incidence with dexlansoprazole than its comparators. (See section 7 Safety Summary) To manage this potential risk, a post-marketing study and labeling recommendations are advised."

DUE TO THE concern of bone fractures, Kapidex was required to conduct a post-marketing clinical trial:

"A CLINICAL TRIAL TO evaluate the effect of Kapidex (dexlansoprazole) Delayed-Release Capsules on bone homeostasis. The primary endpoint will be biomarkers of bone formation and bone resorption. Treatments will include placebo, dexlansoprazole, and esomeprazole (Nexium).

The timetable you submitted on January 12, 2009, states that you will conduct this trial according to the following timetable:

Final Protocol Submission: August 31, 2009

Trial Start Date: October 31, 2009

Final Report Submission: December 31, 2011 "

*AS OF THE writing this book in November 2018 the results of the clinical trial have not been released, and the FDA website shows "No Results Posted."[3]

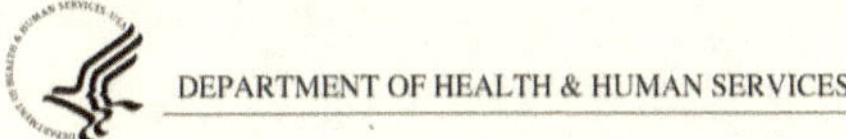

DEPARTMENT OF HEALTH & HUMAN SERVICES

Public Health Service

Food and Drug Administration
Rockville, MD 20857

NDA 22-287

NDA APPROVAL

Takeda Global Research and Development Center, Inc
Attention: Nancianne Knipfer, Ph.D., RAC
Manager, Regulatory Affairs Strategy
One Takeda Parkway
Deerfield, IL 60015

Dear Dr. Knipfer:

Please refer to your new drug application (NDA) dated December 28, 2007, received December 28, 2007, submitted under section 505(b) of the Federal Food, Drug, and Cosmetic Act (FDCA) for Kapidex (dexlansoprazole) Delayed Release Capsules 30, 60, **(b) (4)** mg.

We acknowledge receipt of your submissions dated February 5, 18, 19, 2008; March 7 and 26, 2008; April 28 and 29, 2008; May 22 and 30, 2008; June 24, 26, 30, 2008; July 11 and 15, 2008; August 21 and 26, 2008; September 9, 10, 26, 2008; October 20 and 21, 2008; November 7, 14, 21, 2008; December 10, 17, 23, 2008 and January 12, 13, 14, 22, 23, 27, 28, 2009.

This new drug application provides for the use of Kapidex (dexlansoprazole) Delayed Release Capsules 30 mg for maintaining healing of erosive esophagitis, and for treating heartburn associated with non-erosive gastroesophageal reflux disease (GERD). This new drug application also provides for the use of Kapidex (dexlansoprazole) Delayed Release Capsules 60 mg for healing of all grades of erosive esophagitis.

As discussed in the November 5, 2008 teleconference, we are not approving the **(b) (4)** dose of Kapidex (dexlansoprazole) Delayed Release Capsules.

We have completed our review of this application, as amended. It is approved for the 30 and 60 mg doses, effective on the date of this letter, for use as recommended in the enclosed agreed-upon labeling text.

REQUIRED PEDIATRIC ASSESSMENTS

Under the Pediatric Research Equity Act (PREA) (21 U.S.C. 355c), all applications for new active ingredients, new indications, new dosage forms, new dosing regimens, or new routes of administration are required to contain an assessment of the safety and effectiveness of the product for the claimed indications in pediatric patients unless this requirement is waived, deferred, or inapplicable.

NDA 22-287
Page 2

We are waiving the pediatric study requirement for ages birth to less than one month for the following indications: healing and maintenance of healing of all grades of erosive esophagitis (EE) and treating heartburn associated with non-erosive gastroesophageal reflux disease (GERD) because the necessary studies are impossible or highly impractical.

We are waiving the pediatric study requirement for ages 1-11 months for the following indications: healing and maintenance of healing of all grades of erosive esophagitis (EE) because necessary studies are impossible or highly impractical. The number of pediatric patients with erosive esophagitis in this age group would be limited.

We are deferring submission of your pediatric studies for ages 1 year to 17 years for healing and maintenance of healing of all grades of erosive esophagitis (EE) and for 1 month to 17 years for treating heartburn associated with non-erosive gastroesophageal disease (GERD) because this product is ready for approval for use in adults and the pediatric studies have not been completed.

Your deferred pediatric studies required by section 505B(a) of the Federal Food, Drug, and Cosmetic Act are required postmarketing studies. The status of these postmarketing studies must be reported annually according to 21 CFR 314.81 and section 505B(a)(3)(B) of the Federal Food, Drug, and Cosmetic Act. These required studies are listed below.

1. Deferred pediatric study under PREA for healing and maintenance of healing of all grades of erosive esophagitis (EE) in pediatric patients 1 year to 11 years.

   Final report submission: October 31, 2013

2. Deferred pediatric study under PREA for healing and maintenance of healing of all grades of erosive esophagitis (EE) in pediatric patients 12 years to 17 years.

   Final report submission: March 31, 2013

3. Deferred pediatric study under PREA for treating heartburn associated with non-erosive GERD in pediatric patients aged 1 month to 11 months.

   Final report submission: July 31, 2016

4. Deferred pediatric study under PREA for treating heartburn associated with non-erosive GERD in pediatric patients aged 1 year to 11 years.

   Final report submission: October 31, 2013

5. Deferred pediatric study under PREA for treating heartburn associated with non-erosive GERD in pediatric patients aged 12 years to 17 years.

   Final report submission: March 31, 2013

Submit final study reports to your NDA 22-287. Use the following designator to prominently label all submissions:

Required Pediatric Assessments

NDA 22-287
Page 3

POSTMARKETING REQUIREMENTS UNDER 505(o)

Title IX, Subtitle A, Section 901 of the Food and Drug Administration Amendments Act of 2007 (FDAAA) amends the FDCA to authorize FDA to require holders of approved drug and biological product applications to conduct postmarketing studies and clinical trials for certain purposes, if FDA makes certain findings required by the statute (section 505(o)(3)(A), 21 U.S.C. 355(o)(3)(A)). This provision took effect on March 25, 2008.

We have determined that an analysis of spontaneous postmarketing adverse events reported under subsection 505(k)(1) of the FDCA will not be sufficient to assess a signal of a serious risk for bone fractures in patients who have prolonged use and/or higher doses of Kapidex (dexlansoprazole) Delayed Release Capsules.

Furthermore, the new pharmacovigilance system that FDA is required to establish under section 505(k)(3) of the FDCA has not yet been established and is not sufficient to assess this serious risk.

Finally, we have determined that only a clinical trial (rather than a nonclinical or observational study) will be sufficient to assess this serious risk.

Therefore, based on appropriate scientific data, FDA has determined that you are required, pursuant to section 505(o)(3) of the FDCA, to conduct the following postmarketing clinical trial:

6. A clinical trial to evaluate the effect of Kapidex (dexlansoprazole) Delayed Release Capsules on bone homeostasis. The primary endpoint will be biomarkers of bone formation and bone resorption. Treatments will include: placebo, dexlansoprazole and esomeprazole.

The timetable you submitted on January 12, 2009, states that you will conduct this trial according to the following timetable:

Final protocol Submission:	August 31, 2009
Trial Start Date:	October 31, 2009
Final Report Submission:	December 31, 2011

Submit the protocol to your IND 69,927, with a cross-reference letter to this NDA 22-287. Submit all final reports to your NDA 22-287. Use the following designators to prominently label all submissions, including supplements, relating to this postmarketing clinical trial as appropriate:

- **Required Postmarketing Protocol under 505(o)**
- **Required Postmarketing Final Report under 505(o)**
- **Required Postmarketing Correspondence under 505(o)**

Section 505(o)(3)(E)(ii) of the FDCA requires you to report periodically on the status of any study or clinical trial required under this section. This section also requires you to periodically report to FDA on the status of any study or clinical trial otherwise undertaken to investigate a safety issue. Section 506B of the FDCA, as well as 21 CFR 314.81(b)(2)(vii) requires you to

NDA 22-287
Page 4

report annually on the status of any postmarketing commitments or required studies or clinical trials.

FDA will consider the submission of your annual report under section 506B and 21 CFR 314.81(b)(2)(vii) to satisfy the periodic reporting requirement under section 505(o)(3)(E)(ii) provided that you include the elements listed in 505(o) and 21 CFR 314.81(b)(2(vii). We remind you that to comply with 505(o), your annual report must also include a report on the status of any study or clinical trial otherwise undertaken to investigate a safety issue. Failure to submit an annual report for studies or clinical trials required under 505(o) on the date required will be considered a violation of FDCA section 505(o)(3)(E)(ii) and could result in enforcement action.

CONTENT OF LABELING

As soon as possible, but no later than 14 days from the date of this letter, please submit the content of labeling [21 CFR 314.50(l)] in structured product labeling (SPL) format as described at http://www.fda.gov/oc/datacouncil/spl.html that is identical to the enclosed labeling (text for the package insert, text for the patient package insert). Upon receipt, we will transmit that version to the National Library of Medicine for public dissemination. For administrative purposes, please designate this submission, "SPL for approved NDA 22-287."

CARTON AND IMMEDIATE CONTAINER LABELS

Submit final printed carton and container labels that are identical to the January 13, 2009 submitted carton and immediate container labels, with the exception of the Hospital Unit Dose Blister Labels for 30 mg and 60 mg doses, of which we accept the January 23, 2009 submission as soon as they are available, but no more than 30 days after they are printed. Please submit these labels electronically according to the guidance for industry titled *Providing Regulatory Submissions in Electronic Format – Human Pharmaceutical Product Applications and Related Submissions Using the eCTD Specifications (October 2005)*. Alternatively, you may submit 12 paper copies, with 6 of the copies individually mounted on heavy-weight paper or similar material. For administrative purposes, designate this submission **"Final Printed Carton and Container Labels for approved NDA 22-287"**. Approval of this submission by FDA is not required before the labeling is used.

Marketing the product(s) with FPL that is not identical to the approved labeling text may render the product misbranded and an unapproved new drug.

PROMOTIONAL MATERIALS

You may request advisory comments on proposed introductory advertising and promotional labeling. To do so, submit, in triplicate, a cover letter requesting advisory comments, the proposed materials in draft or mock-up form with annotated references, and the package insert(s) to:

NDA 22-281
Page 5

Food and Drug Administration
Center for Drug Evaluation and Research
Division of Drug Marketing, Advertising, and Communications
5901-B Ammendale Road
Beltsville, MD 20705-1266

As required under 21 CFR 314.81(b)(3)(i), you must submit final promotional materials, and the package insert(s), at the time of initial dissemination or publication, accompanied by a Form FDA 2253. For instruction on completing the Form FDA 2253, see page 2 of the Form. For more information about submission of promotional materials to the Division of Drug Marketing, Advertising, and Communications (DDMAC), see www.fda.gov/cder/ddmac.

LETTERS TO HEALTH CARE PROFESSIONALS

If you issue a letter communicating important safety related information about this drug product (i.e., a "Dear Health Care Professional" letter), we request that you submit an electronic copy of the letter to both this NDA and to the following address:

MedWatch
Food and Drug Administration
Suite 12B05
5600 Fishers Lane
Rockville, MD 20857

REPORTING REQUIREMENTS

We remind you that you must comply with reporting requirements for an approved NDA (21 CFR 314.80 and 314.81).

If you have any questions, call Anna Simon, Regulatory Project Manager, at (301) 796-3509.

Sincerely,

{See appended electronic signature page}

Donna Griebel, M.D.
Director
Division of Gastroenterology Products
Office of Drug Evaluation III
Center for Drug Evaluation and Research

Enclosure: Package Insert

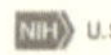 U.S. National Library of Medicine

ClinicalTrials.gov

Effect of Dexlansoprazole on Bone Homeostasis

⚠ The safety and scientific validity of this study is the responsibility of the study sponsor and investigators. Listing a study does not mean it has been evaluated by the U.S. Federal Government. Read our disclaimer for details.

ClinicalTrials.gov Identifier:
NCT01216293

Recruitment Status ❶: Completed
First Posted ❶: October 7, 2010
Last Update Posted ❶: March 3, 2015

Sponsor:
Takeda

Information provided by (Responsible Party):
Takeda

| Study Details | Tabular View | **No Results Posted** | Disclaimer |

How to Read a Study Record

No Study Results Posted on ClinicalTrials.gov for this Study

About Study Results Reporting on ClinicalTrials.gov

Recruitment Status ❶:	Completed
Actual Primary Completion Date ❶:	August 2014
Actual Study Completion Date ❶:	February 2015

5

HIPAA

Before 1996, a patient's medical records were not in a standard format with the ability to be viewed and edited by numerous physicians. Because of the lack of transparency, adverse medical outcomes can occur due to the reduced knowledge between multiple physician offices. A significant issue with pharmaceuticals is their drug to drug interactions which can harm the patient. It is imperative that physicians and pharmacists know what medications the patient is taking to avoid adverse events which could lead to death.

Another issue with non-electronic medical records is the potential for information loss. If the office would endure a fire or other disaster, thousands of patient files could be lost along with years of their medical history. Also, not having a patient's information in a database, could allow for fraud and prescription overuse.

Congress passed the Health Insurance Portability and Accountability Act (HIPAA) in 1996[1]. The final vote in the House of Representatives was 421 - 2 and the final vote in the Senate was 98 - 0. President Clinton signed the Bill into law on August 21, 1996.

HIPAA mandated the establishment of federal standards for patient health information through mandated compliance and strict regulations. The main parts of the law are regarding the protection of health insurance coverage for workers and their families when they change or lose their jobs and Administrative Simplification (AS) provisions. The Administrative Simplification provisions comprise the crucial area of my case.

TITLE II—PREVENTING HEALTH CARE FRAUD AND ABUSE; ADMINISTRATIVE SIMPLIFICATION; MEDICAL LIABILITY REFORM

Title II comprises fraud and abuse controls, data collection, and Administrative Simplifications. The law requires the establishment of national standards for electronic health care transactions, also known as electronic medical records (EMR). Along with EMR, Title II initiated national identifiers for health care providers, health insurance plans, and employers.

EMR has many benefits not only the patient but for the healthcare system as a whole. A patient's EMR consists of past history, the family history which the patient provided, prior diagnosis, previous treatments - ones that worked and ones that didn't, medications, allergies, lab results, immunizations, and any past x-rays or scans.

With all of the information available through multiple patient-physician offices, it is important to keep patient confidentiality. All physician offices are required to inform you of your HIPAA rights and to make sure you acknowledge these rights. It is imperative for the patient to document who is able to see your medical records since if your spouse calls to get information and is not on your list, they will be denied.

Employees of medical offices, as well as sales representatives, have had training on HIPAA and what is allowed to be viewed and what is not. As sales representatives, we are not allowed to look through patients charts or talk about patients by name.

The fact that the court ruled against me for not having actual prescriptions of patients is something that is going to hurt pharmaceutical whistleblowers for years to come. One of the main purposes of HIPAA is to protect patient information, including what medications they are on. How am I expected to obtain prescriptions without going public asking for them? Well, that is what I am doing now!

If you have experienced a broken bone while on Dexilant 60mg I would encourage you to inform your physician and also go to my website, www.appleQD.com, to add yourself to the list. The information you should provide is:

-Your name and contact information including email address

-Dates you took Dexilant

-Dosage strength of Dexilant

-Date and bone broken

6

TAP PHARMACEUTICALS

I started with TAP Pharmaceuticals in December 2002. TAP Pharmaceuticals was short for Takeda Abbott Partnership Pharmaceuticals and was founded in 1977 as a joint venture between Takeda Pharmaceuticals and Abbott Laboratories. The partnership was dissolved in 2008 and TAP Pharmaceuticals was divided between Takeda and Abbott.

The two most successful products sold by TAP were Prevacid and Lupron. The Prevacid and Lupron representatives were divided into separate sales forces since they were for different issues calling on different offices. In 2008 when TAP was dissolved, the gastroenterology division went to Takeda Pharmaceuticals and the Lupron division went to Abbott Laboratories.

In 1977 when the partnership began Takeda did not have sales representatives in the United States. Takeda Pharmaceuticals is a Japanese company dating back to 1781 and is currently the largest pharmaceutical company in Japan and 20th in the world, with annual sales totaling over $16 billion. Takeda eventually created a base of operations and a sales force in the United States. In 1999, Takeda launched the diabetes drug Actos, which will become the best selling diabetes medication in the world, at that time, reaching sales of $4 Billion in 2008 for the U.S. alone. A future chapter will describe Actos and the legal actions against Takeda including their admission to destroying documents in a lawsuit related to bladder cancer.

In 2008 when TAP dissolved, the gastroenterology representatives and leadership were blended with the Takeda Pharmaceuticals North America organization.

The amount of changes in the way we are permitted to promote pharmaceuticals has created a type of false sense of security in the industry. We are aware of the rules and regulations, as well as the penalties that have been paid out in recent years. Every major pharmaceutical company has an Ethics & Compliance department along with human resources employees that handle issues and concerns related to company policy. With so many people involved, how could something slip through? Because it was hiding in plain sight.

I was not the first whistleblower against TAP/Takeda Pharmaceuticals. In 2001 the U.S. Department of Justice, States Attorneys General, and TAP Pharmaceutical Products settled criminal and civil charges against TAP related to federal and state Medicare fraud and illegal marketing of the drug Lupron. TAP plead guilty to conspiracy to violate the Prescription Drug Marketing Act by causing free samples to be illegally billed to the Medicare program. Lupron is an in-office injectable used to treat prostate cancer and infertility. TAP paid a total of $875 million, which was a record high at the time.

Here is the release from the U.S. Department of Justice[1]:

FOR IMMEDIATE RELEASE
   CIV
   WEDNESDAY, OCTOBER 3, 2001
   (202) 514-2007
   WWW.USDOJ.GOV

TDD (202) 514-1888

TAP PHARMACEUTICAL PRODUCTS INC. AND SEVEN OTHERS CHARGED WITH HEALTH CARE CRIMES; COMPANY AGREES TO PAY $875 MILLION TO SETTLE CHARGES

BOSTON, MA... United States Attorney Michael J. Sullivan, Department of Health and Human Services Inspector General Janet Rehnquist, Assistant Inspector General for Investigations and Director of the Department of Defense Criminal Investigation Service Carol Levy, and Special Agent in Charge of the Federal Bureau of Investigation in New England Charles S. Prouty, announced today that:

(1) TAP PHARMACEUTICAL PRODUCTS INC. ("TAP"), a major American pharmaceutical manufacturer, has agreed to pay $875,000,000 to resolve criminal charges and civil liabilities in connection with its fraudulent drug pricing and marketing conduct with regard to Lupron, a drug sold by TAP primarily for treatment of advanced prostate cancer in men. The global agreement includes:

(a) TAP has agreed to plead guilty to a conspiracy to violate the PrescriptionDrug Marketing Act and to pay a $290,000,000 criminal fine, the largest criminal fine ever in a health care fraud prosecution. The plea agreement between the United States and TAP specifically states that TAP's criminal conduct caused losses of $145,000,000.

(b) TAP has agreed to settle its federal civil False Claims Act liabilities and to pay the U.S. Government $559,483,560 for filing false and fraudulent claims with the Medicare and Medicaid programs as a result of TAP's fraudulent drug pricing schemes and sales and marketing misconduct.

(c) TAP has agreed to settle its civil liabilities to the fifty states and the District of Columbia and to pay them $25,516,440 for filing false and fraudulent claims with the states, as a result of TAP's drug pricing and marketing misconduct, and from TAP's failure to provide the state Medicaid programs TAP's best price for those drugs as required by law.

(d) TAP has agreed to comply with the terms of a sweeping corporate integrity agreement which, among other things, significantly changes the manner in which TAP supervises its marketing and sales staff, and ensures that TAP will report to the Medicare and Medicaid programs the true average sale price for drugs reimbursed by those programs.

(2) A federal grand jury returned an indictment unsealed today, charging one physician and six TAP managers with conspiracy to pay kickbacks to doctors and other customers, conspiracy to defraud the state Medicaid programs on TAP's obligation to sell products to those programs at its best price, and conspiracy to violate the Prescription Drug Marketing Act by causing free samples to be illegally billed to the Medicare program. The indictment charges that the TAP defendants offered to give things of value, including free drugs, so-called educational grants, trips to resorts, free consulting services, medical equipment, and forgiveness of debt, to physicians and other customers to obtain their referrals of prescriptions for Lupron to Medicare program beneficiaries, in violation of the anti-kickback statute. The indictment also charges that the TAP defendants aided and abetted, and caused the billings to hundreds of elderly Medicare program beneficiaries and to the Medicare program directly, for thousands of free samples of Lupron, used in the treatment of prostate cancer, in violation of the Prescription Drug Marketing Act.

The seven individuals charged in the indictment unsealed today are:

(1) ALAN MACKENZIE, age 49, of 27068 Wellington Court, Barrington, Illinois, and formerly Vice President of Sales for TAP.

(2) JANICE SWIRSKI, age 40, of 6 Bellingham Drive, Chestnut Hill, Massachusetts, and formerly a National Account Manager with TAP.

(3) HENRY VAN MOURICK, age 43, of 23 Golfwood Court, Roseville, California, and currently a District Manager employed by TAP.

(4) DONNA TOM, age 37, of 141 East 56th Street, New York, New York, and formerly a District Manager employed by TAP.

(5) KIMBERLEE CHASE, age 35, of 108 Dedham Street, Dover, Massachusetts, and formerly a District Manager employed by TAP.

(6) DAVID GUIDO, age 30, of 131 New London Road, Colchester, Connecticut, and currently a Hospital Account Executive employed by TAP.

(7) DR. JOHN ROMANO, age 48, of 110 Long Pond Road, Plymouth, Massachusetts, an urologist with a practice in Plymouth, Massachusetts.

Prior to yesterday's indictment, four other physicians have been charged and have pleaded guilty in this investigation: Dr. Rodney Mannion, a urologist practicing in LaPorte and Michigan City, Indiana, was charged on February 28, 2000 with healthcare fraud. Dr. Mannion pleaded guilty to that charge on April 25, 2000. Dr. Jacob Zamstein, a urologist practicing in Bloomfield, Connecticut, was charged on November 3, 2000 with healthcare fraud and pleaded guilty on December 27, 2000. Dr. Joseph Spinella, a urologist practicing in Bristol, Connecticut, was charged on December 8, 2000 with healthcare fraud and pleaded guilty on March 29, 2001. Dr. Joel Olstein, a urologist practicing in Lewiston, Maine, was charged on April 11, 2001 with healthcare fraud and pleaded guilty on July 18, 2001.

Lupron is marketed by TAP primarily for the treatment of prostate cancer. Lupron is identical in effectiveness to the drug Zolodex, produced by a competitor, which was also available for prescription in the 1990s. While Medicare does not pay for most drugs needed by Medicare beneficiaries, Medicare does cover drugs, such as Lupron, that must be injected under the supervision of a physician. Medicare paid for 80% of either the urologist's charge for Lupron or the average wholesale price reported by TAP, whichever was lower, and the patient was responsible for the remaining 20% as a copayment.

As part of its civil allegations, the Government alleged that throughout the1990s, TAP set and controlled the price at which the Medicare program reimbursed physicians for the prescription of Lupron by reporting its average wholesale price ("AWP"). The AWP reported by TAP was significantly higher than the average sales price TAP offered physicians and other customers for the drug. The Government alleged that TAP marketed the spread between its discounted prices paid by physicians and the significantly higher Medicare reimbursement based on AWP as an inducement to physicians to obtain their Lupron business. The Government further alleged that TAP concealed the true discounted prices paid by physicians from Medicare, and falsely advised physicians to report the higher AWP rather than their real discounted price for the drug. The Government further alleged that TAP set its AWPs of Lupron at levels far higher than the price for which wholesalers or distributors actually sold the drug, resulting in falsely inflated prices that were neither the physician's actual cost nor the true wholesaler's average price.

"The Medicare and Medicaid drug programs are bulwarks against the financial hardship that can be caused by the need for life-saving medical treatments," said Robert D. McCallum, Jr., Assistant Attorney General for the Justice Department's Civil Division. "These programs cannot afford abuses that enrich doctors or drug companies at the expense of taxpayers and patients. This settlement agreement and the compliance steps that TAP has agreed to take will reinforce the government's long-standing objective of paying Medicare and Medicaid providers for the reasonable costs of the drugs they administer."

"The urologists and the TAP employees who knowingly participated in this broad conspiracy took advantage of older Americans suffering from prostate cancer. The indictment unsealed today alleges that TAP employees sought to influence the doctors' decisions about what drug to prescribe to patients by giving them kickbacks and bribes, from free samples to free consulting services to expensive trips to golf and ski resorts to so-called educational grants," said U.S. Attorney Sullivan. "In all instances where the kickbacks worked to ensure the prescription of TAP's product Lupron, the Medicare Program and the elderly Americans suffering from prostate cancer paid more for their care than if the doctor had prescribed the competitor's product."

"Medicare beneficiaries and all American patients need to get the right pharmaceuticals, based on medical criteria, and at a fair price. This is crucial both to ensure good quality health care and to use our resources effectively. Today's settlement is a clear message that the federal government will protect the best interests of beneficiaries and taxpayers," said HHS Secretary Tommy G. Thompson.

"This prosecution has resulted in the largest criminal and civil recoveries in any health care fraud case in the country. The fraud schemes used by TAP Pharmaceuticals and others impacts significantly on the integrity of TRICARE, the Department of Defense's healthcare system," stated DCIS Special Agent in Charge Edward Bradley. "Healthcare fraud increases patients' costs and negatively effects the delivery of health care services to over 8 million military members, retirees, and their dependents."

The indictment unsealed today against the seven individuals alleges that inducements to physicians included free products; free consulting services; trips to expensive golf and ski resorts;

money disguised as "educational grants," but in fact was used and intended to be used for many purposes, including cocktail party bar tabs, office Christmas parties, medical equipment, travel expenses for urologists and their staff to attend conferences; and discounts on Lupron sold to treat endometriosis in women to effect a lower price on Lupron used in the treatment of men with prostate cancer.

The investigation commenced in the District of Massachusetts in 1997 after a urologist employed by Tufts Associated Health Maintenance Organization ("Tufts HMO") in Waltham, Dr. Joseph Gerstein, reported to law enforcement authorities that he had been offered an educational grant if he would reverse a decision he had made on behalf of Tufts that it would only cover the less expensive drug Zoladex. As charged in the indictment, SWIRSKI and CHASE met with Dr. Gerstein after he began working with the FBI and the Office of Inspector General, and during those meetings, offered him $65,000 in educational grants that he could use for any purpose "whatever," together with discounts on other products, if he would reverse Tufts' decision not to include Lupron on its formulary for treating patients that it insured who were suffering from prostate cancer. The investigation was also triggered by a civil False Claims Act suit filed in 1996 by Douglas Durand, after he had quit his employment at TAP as Vice President of Sales, after just one year because of his concerns about the illegal marketing conduct of some of TAP's employees.

The civil False Claims Act provides that where persons submit, cause others to submit, or conspire to submit, false or fraudulent claims to the United States Government, including its federal health care programs, the Government is entitled to recover treble damages and $5,500 to $11,000 for each false or fraudulent claim submitted. Private individuals, like Dr. Gerstein and Douglas Durand, are allowed to file whistleblower suits under the False Claims Act to bring the government information about wrongdoing, and if the government is successful in resolving or litigating their claims, to share in the recovery by receiving generally 15% to 25% of the amount recovered. As a part of today's resolution, those two individuals together with Tufts Associated HMO will share as whistleblowers, pursuant to the Congressional directive in the False Claims Act, 17% of the civil recovery, or an amount of approximately $95 million.

"The payment by TAP of nearly $900 million including the highest criminal fine ever imposed on any health care company, and the indictment of the six TAP employees sends a very strong signal to the pharmaceutical industry that it best police its employees' conduct and deal strongly with those who would gain sales at the expense of the health care programs for the poor and the elderly and the persons insured by those programs," said U.S. Attorney Sullivan.

As part of a condition for doing business in the future with providers who are members of the Medicare and Medicaid programs, TAP agreed to enter into an extensive Corporate Integrity Agreement. That agreement provides for significant training of TAP's sales and marketing employees and changes in supervision and controls. It also requires TAP to report to the Medicare and Medicaid programs accurate pricing information showing TAP's true average sales price.

"In recent years, the pharmaceutical industry has come under increasing scrutiny for its pricing, sales, and marketing practices. The OIG, together with other government agencies, will use all available enforcement authorities, where appropriate, to address these practices," said HHS Inspector General Janet Rehnquist.

The entire amount of the $290 million criminal fine paid by TAP will go to the Department of Justice's Crime Victims Fund. The Fund was established in 1984 by the Victims of Crime Act ("VOCA") and serves as a major funding source for victim services throughout the country. Each year, millions of dollars are deposited into this fund from criminal fines, forfeited bail bonds, penalty fees, and special assessments collected by U.S. Attorney's Offices, U.S. Courts, and the Bureau of Prisons. State assistance programs use VOCA funds to provide or contract for services to victims of rape, drunk driving, child abuse, domestic violence, homicide, and other crimes. Victims of federal, as well as state crimes, are eligible to receive VOCA-funded services.

The investigation is continuing.

The investigation has been conducted by the agents from the Federal Bureau of Investigation, the Office of Investigations for the Office of Inspector General for the Department of Health and Human Services, the Food and Drug Administration's Office of Criminal Investigations and the Department of Defense's Defense Criminal Investigation Service. On the criminal side, the investigation and prosecution are being handled by Assistant U.S. Attorney Michael K. Loucks, Health Care Fraud Chief. On the civil side, the investigation and prosecution are being handled by Assistant U.S. Attorney Susan Winkler, assisted by Department of Justice Trial Attorney T. Reed Stephens. The Corporate Integrity Agreement was negotiated by Office of General Counsel, Office of Inspector General Assistant Counsel Mary Riordan.

Press Contact: Samantha Martin, (617) 748-3139

Doug Durand was the Vice-President of Sales at TAP Pharmaceuticals when he became a whistleblower in 1995. He was the first to file the illegal marketing conduct and, when the settlement was paid, he walked away with $77 million. From the settlement, TAP agreed to perform annual Corporate Integrity Agreement training for all of its employees on Ethics and Compliance issues.

I applied for and was part of the initial G-Force specialty representative team. Our role was to overlap entire primary care districts and concentrate on gastroenterologists, ENT's, rheumatologists, and specific high volume primary care offices. We would share the specialty offices with the primary care representatives we overlapped geographically while taking point on specific programs and promotions.

Kapidex (Dexilant) was approved by the FDA on January 30, 2009. In our training for Dexilant, we only talked about and promoted the 60mg dose. Our primary promotional pieces, as well as the only samples given, were 60mg. It is vital with a new product to instruct the physicians on how to write the prescriptions, and we were told to educate our physicians to write 60mg. Our marketing material had a sample prescription pad on it to show the correct way to prescribe Dexilant, and you guessed it, 60mg. We were instructed to promote Dexilant 60mg for GERD, and we did so without thinking twice about it. GERD stands for GastroEsophageal Reflux Disorder, heartburn for the everyday person.

Common everyday heartburn, like the type you get after eating a spicy meal, then goes away, is not GERD. According to the Mayo Clinic[2], GERD is defined as mild acid reflux that occurs at least twice a week or a moderate to severe acid reflux that happens at least once a week. Transient relaxations of the lower esophageal sphincter allow stomach acid to "reflux" up into the esophagus causing pain and discomfort. Common signs of GERD are heartburn, chest pain, difficulty swallowing, regurgitation, and the sensation of a lump in your throat.

The FDA approved indications for Dexilant are Erosive Esophagitis for 8 weeks at 60mg, maintaining healed erosive esophagitis at 30mg, and GERD at 30mg.[3] To diagnose Erosive Esophagitis, an endoscopy needs to be performed by a trained physician, usually a gastroenterologist. Yet we were promoting Dexilant to primary care physicians and instructing them to give 60mg samples and to write for the same 60mg. I can keep going on about the 60mg, but my point is we never talked about the

30mg dose even though we should have. The issue would be different if the patient tried the 30mg dose for a month and it wasn't enough medicine to control the patient's heartburn so they were increased to the 60mg dose, but that wasn't the case.

As acknowledged by the President and CEO of Takeda Pharmaceuticals North America in a letter dated November 19, 2009, Mr. Shinji Honda stated, "Kapidex is building on Takeda's established presence in the PPI market. For more than a year, Takeda has been refocusing promotion, sales and sampling efforts to Kapidex." We were able to use our relationships, made by promoting Prevacid, to leverage our Dexilant sales and it worked exceptionally well. No one talked about negative issues only how much better the patients can feel on Dexilant with its Dual Delayed Release. The Dual Delayed Release is from different coatings on the granules in the capsule. Twenty-five percent of the granules are for immediate release, and seventy-five percent will be released four to five hours later when the pH changes as the granules move through the stomach and into the small intestine.

Our Dexilant sales were strong, and I was at the top of my region for the first three quarters of the year. Remember what I said earlier about how important a strong launch is to get the refills along with new patients, I did it well. It wasn't until several months after the Dexilant launch that I realized the 60mg promotion issue and what to do about it. I knew all of the details about Dexilant, but the problem was hiding in plain sight.

There are always people who will blindly do what is asked of them. Sometimes they aren't aware of what they are doing is wrong, and sometimes they just don't care. I will give my fellow ex-coworkers the benefit of the doubt, since, why would we think the company would be so blatant about it if it were wrong? Talk about hiding in plain sight. If I didn't know the history of Dexilant, that they initially wanted 90mg and 60mg, I am not sure how long, if ever, it would have taken me to figure it out.

In the book "GRIT – The Power of Passion and Perseverance" by Angela Duckworth[4] she refers to a parable about three workers building a church that stuck with me. When asked what they do, the first worker replied that he has a job as a bricklayer. The second worker replied that he is a bricklayer constructing a building. The third worker said that he is a bricklayer building a house of God. The bricklayers viewed what they do as a job, a career, and a calling.

To take this one step further, which was not the author's intention, but imagine how the third worker, who saw laying bricks for the church as a calling, would feel if he discovered that the foreman used lower standard materials to increase profits. Now imagine, what if by using the lower quality materials a safety issue arose seriously injuring worshippers during a wedding or funeral service. How does that change how you feel?

7

PREVACID

Prevacid (lansoprazole) was approved in the United States in 1995 as the second proton pump inhibitor (PPI) after Prilosec. Over the following years, Prevacid earned a total of 13 indications and dosage forms including a capsule, a solutab (dissolving oral tablet), and an intravenous form. Prevacid received approved indications for pediatric use down to 1 year of age.

After gaining extensions through new indications, new formulations, and pediatric use, Prevacid's patent protection expired in November 2009. As stated in a Securities and Exchange Commission filing,[1] Prevacid "is one of the top five prescription brands in the US in terms of total prescription dollar sales. The drug achieved $3.37 billion in annual sales in the US in 2008." That was a big financial hole to fill and a lot of pressure for the sales force to accomplish. The three indications for Dexilant were three of the thirteen that Prevacid has, along with the same mechanism of action. They are both Proton Pump Inhibitors (PPI's) indicated for gastroesophageal reflux disease (GERD), erosive esophagitis (EE), and maintaining healed erosive esophagitis.

PPI's work by specific inhibition of the (H+, K+)-ATPase enzyme system at the secretory surface of the parietal cell. Shutting down the parietal cells reduces the amount of gastric acid that can be produced in the stomach. Parietal cells die off and are replaced by new ones on a regular basis, needing another dose of medication to keep the gastric acid production under control.

Some patients produce too much gastric acid, and some patients might be more sensitive to the burning sensation of gastric acid than others. The main reason for heartburn is from transient relaxations of the lower esophageal sphincter, which allows for gastric acid to cause discomfort and possible damage to the esophagus. The lower esophageal sphincter is a junction between your lower esophagus and the stomach. It opens and closes to allow food and liquids to enter the stomach without coming back up. At times material can be pushed back up such as if you bend over and put pressure on your stomach virtually squeezing it causing the contents to move. Carbonated drinks can also cause reflux due to the added gas in the contained area of the stomach.

Takeda planned to use the Prevacid name recognition to build Dexilant sales. The last Prevacid samples were given out in January 2009 and replaced with Dexilant 60mg. The Prevacid.com website had Dexilant information on it as well as a link to the Dexilant.com website.

Prevacid had great recognition and physicians loved it. When I began working at TAP Pharmaceuticals, it was my only product, and I grew to know Prevacid exceptionally well. We had marketing pieces, medical journal articles, and television advertisements to help us in our sales. On top of that, the insurance coverage was fantastic along with a great coupon program.

8

DEXILANT

Dexilant (dexlansoprazole) was launched in 2009 under the brand name Kapidex. The name was changed from Kapidex to Dexilant due to some issues at the pharmacy level with a similar sounding medication. Dexilant comes in a 30mg and a 60mg dose although for an extended period of time the 30mg was not sampled and many physicians were not aware it was an option.

A brief overview of Dexilant is that it is the R-enantiomer of Prevacid (lansoprazole). To keep it simple, think of your left and right hands, they mirror each other but are not the same. Think of Dexilant as the right hand of Prevacid along with a dual delayed release (DDR) technology to make one pill work as two. The DDR refers to the coating on the granules inside the Dexilant capsule. In each capsule there are two different types of granules, one for immediate release and another to be released several hours later based on pH levels in the small intestine. It works similar to a patient taking a pill, then taking another pill several hours later, but is more patient-friendly since there is no risk of missing the second dose. The right-handed enantiomer of

Prevacid is considered a new drug with a new patent life. It is thought to improve bioavailability and metabolism, and the efficiency of inhibiting the proton pump function of the parietal cell. Parietal cells are what produce gastric (stomach) acid and by shutting them down reduces the amount of acid in the stomach which reduces heartburn in the patient. Basically, it is thought to work better. In the Dexilant package insert (PI), it states "initial U.S. approval 1995 (lansoprazole)" but it was still given a new patent.

With a $3 billion a year medicine, Prevacid, going off patent, Takeda had a lot of pressure to switch those patients over to Dexilant. As stated by the President and CEO of Takeda Pharmaceuticals North America, Inc., Shinji Honda in a letter from November 19, 2009:

"With loss of patent exclusivity for Prevacid earlier this month, Prevacid sales are expected to continue to experience a significant drop for this fiscal year - approximately 30 percent year-over-year compared to sales results FY2008. Over the years, Prevacid has been a significant contributor to Takeda's overall sales. To continue with the legacy established by Prevacid, we are employing a combination of strategies to provide continued value from this important product to Takeda and to the patients that rely on Prevacid. In its generic and OTC forms, Prevacid will continue to meet the needs of patients and providers. Additionally, Kapidex is building on Takeda's established presence in the PPI market. For more than a year, Takeda has been refocusing promotion, sales and sampling efforts to Kapidex. Again, I want to thank the numerous individuals who helped make Prevacid one of the best selling prescription medications in the United States."

THE FOLLOWING IS from the U.S. Department of Health and

Human Services New Drug Application (NDA) Letter requiring Takeda to conduct a study on patients in the general population after the approval of Dexilant. Information from clinical trials has limitations due to the relatively low number of subjects. Once the medication is approved and marketed to physicians the number of patients increases dramatically. With this increase, adverse events are known to show up that were not present during the clinical trials. With mixed reviews by the FDA investigators, Dexilant was approved but with the stipulation that a post-marketing study will assess the bone fracture concern.[1]

POSTMARKETING REQUIREMENTS UNDER 505(o)

TITLE IX, Subtitle A, Section 901 of the Food and Drug Administration Amendments Act of 2007 (FDAAA) amends the FDCA to authorize FDA to require holders of approved drug and biological product applications to conduct postmarketing studies and clinical trials for certain purposes, if FDA makes certain findings required by the statute (section 505(o)(3)(A), 21 U.S.C. 355(o)(3)(A)). This provision took effect on March 25, 2008.

We have determined that an analysis of spontaneous postmarketing adverse events reported under subsection 505(k)(1) of the FDCA will not be sufficient to assess a signal of a serious risk for bone fractures in patients who have prolonged use and/or higher doses of Kapidex (dexlansoprazole) Delayed Release Capsules.

Furthermore, the new pharmacovigilance system that FDA is required to establish under section 505(k)(3) of the FDCA has not yet been established and is not sufficient to assess this serious risk.

Finally, we have determined that only a clinical trial (rather than a nonclinical or observational study) will be sufficient to assess this serious risk.

Therefore, based on appropriate scientific data, FDA has determined that you are required, pursuant to section 505(o)(3) of the FDCA, to conduct the following postmarketing clinical trial:

6. A clinical trial to evaluate the effect of Kapidex (dexlansoprazole) Delayed Release Capsules on bone homeostasis. The primary endpoint will be biomarkers of bone formation and bone resorption. Treatments will include: placebo, dexlansoprazole and esomeprazole.

The timetable you submitted on January 12, 2009, states that you will conduct this trial according to the following timetable:

Final protocol Submission: August 31, 2009

Trial Start Date: October 31, 2009

Final Report Submission: December 31, 2011

Submit the protocol to your IND 69,927, with a cross-reference letter to this NDA 22-287. Submit all final reports to your NDA 22-287. Use the following designators to prominently label all submissions, including supplements, relating to this postmarketing clinical trial as appropriate:

¥Required Postmarketing Protocol under 505(o)

¥Required Postmarketing Final Report under 505(o)

¥Required Postmarketing Correspondence under 505(o)

Section 505(o)(3)(E)(ii) of the FDCA requires you to report periodically on the status of any study or clinical trial required under this section. This section also requires you to periodically report to FDA on the status of any study or clinical trial otherwise undertaken to investigate a safety issue. Section 506B of the FDCA, as well as 21 CFR 314.81(b)(2)(vii) requires you to report annually on the status of any postmarketing commitments or required studies or clinical trials.

FDA will consider the submission of your annual report under section 506B and 21 CFR 314.81(b)(2)(vii) to satisfy the periodic reporting requirement under section 505(o)(3)(E)(ii) provided that you include the elements listed in 505(o) and 21 CFR 314.81(b)(2(vii). We remind you that to comply with 505(o), your annual report must also include a report on the status of any study or clinical trial otherwise undertaken to investigate a safety issue. Failure to submit an annual report for studies or clinical trials required under 505(o) on the date required will be considered a violation of FDCA section 505(o)(3)(E)(ii) and could result in enforcement action.

IT IS important to note that the Approval of Kapidex/Dexilant was contingent on Takeda starting and completing this post-marketing study to determine the effect of Dexilant on bone fractures. The letter stated its concern that the analysis of reported adverse events from patients is not enough because not every patient is expected to report their adverse events.

According to the U.S. Food and Drug Administration, "an adverse event is any undesirable experience associated with the use of a medical product in a patient. The event is serious and should be reported to the FDA when the patient outcome is: Death, Life-threatening, Hospitalization (initial or prolonged), Disability or Permanent Damage, Congenital Anomaly/Birth Defect, Required Intervention to Prevent Permanent Impairment or Other Serious Events."[2]

The typical adverse events we see are those that happen to greater than two percent of the patients during the study. This data is collected from everyone in the study including patients taking placebo to determine if the active drug is causing the concern. During the study, patients are encouraged to report everything that could be considered an adverse event.

The biggest adverse events for Dexilant during the clinical trials were:

Diarrhea 4.8%

Abdominal Pain 4.0%

Nausea 2.9%

Since the main reporting of adverse events are during the clinical trials, which consist of only a few thousand people, or less, a lot of negative feedback doesn't come to light until the drug has been on the market for a few years.

"WE HAVE DETERMINED that an analysis of spontaneous post marketing adverse events reported under subsection 505(k)(1) of the FDCA will not be sufficient to assess a signal of a serious risk for bone fractures in patients who have prolonged use and/or higher doses of Kapidex (dexlansoprazole) Delayed Release Capsules."

"FINALLY, we have determined that only a clinical trial (rather than a nonclinical or observational study) will be sufficient to assess this serious risk."

"THEREFORE, based on appropriate scientific data, FDA has determined that you are required, pursuant to section 505(o)(3) of the FDCA, to conduct the following postmarketing clinical trial:"

"6. A clinical trial to evaluate the effect of Kapidex (dexlansoprazole) Delayed Release Capsules on bone homeostasis. The primary endpoint will be biomarkers of bone formation and bone resorption. Treatments will include: placebo, dexlansoprazole and esomeprazole."

.   .   .

"THE TIMETABLE you submitted on January 12, 2009, states that you will conduct this trial according to the following timetable:"

FINAL PROTOCOL SUBMISSION: August 31, 2009
   Trial Start Date:October 31, 2009
   Final Report Submission:December 31, 2011

ACCORDING to clinicaltrials.gov
   https://clinicaltrials.gov/ct2/show/results/NCT01216293

THE STUDY WAS STARTED in January 2011 and completed in August 2014. The actual study completion was in February 2015 and the last update on the government website was on March 3, 2015.[3]

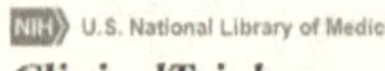

ClinicalTrials.gov

Effect of Dexlansoprazole on Bone Homeostasis

⚠ The safety and scientific validity of this study is the responsibility of the study sponsor and investigators. Listing a study does not mean it has been evaluated by the U.S. Federal Government. Read our disclaimer for details.

ClinicalTrials.gov Identifier:
NCT01216293

Recruitment Status ❶: Completed
First Posted ❶: October 7, 2010
Last Update Posted ❶: March 3, 2015

Sponsor:
Takeda

Information provided by (Responsible Party):
Takeda

| **Study Details** | Tabular View | No Results Posted | Disclaimer |

How to Read a Study Record

Study Description   Go to ▾

Brief Summary:
The purpose of this study is to evaluate the effect of dexlansoprazole modified release (MR), once daily (QD), on bone homeostasis.

Condition or disease ❶	Intervention/treatment ❶	Phase ❶
Homeostasis	Drug: Dexlansoprazole	Phase 1
Bone and Bones	Drug: Esomeprazole	
	Drug: Placebo	

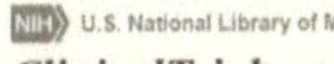

ClinicalTrials.gov

Effect of Dexlansoprazole on Bone Homeostasis

⚠ The safety and scientific validity of this study is the responsibility of the study sponsor and investigators. Listing a study does not mean it has been evaluated by the U.S. Federal Government. Read our disclaimer for details.

ClinicalTrials.gov Identifier:
NCT01216293

Recruitment Status ❶: Completed
First Posted ❶: October 7, 2010
Last Update Posted ❶: March 3, 2015

Sponsor:
Takeda

Information provided by (Responsible Party):
Takeda

| Study Details | **Tabular View** | No Results Posted | Disclaimer |

How to Read a Study Record

Tracking Information

First Submitted Date [ICMJE]	October 5, 2010
First Posted Date [ICMJE]	October 7, 2010
Last Update Posted Date	March 3, 2015
Study Start Date [ICMJE]	January 2011
Actual Primary Completion Date	August 2014 (Final data collection date for primary outcome measure)
Current Primary Outcome	

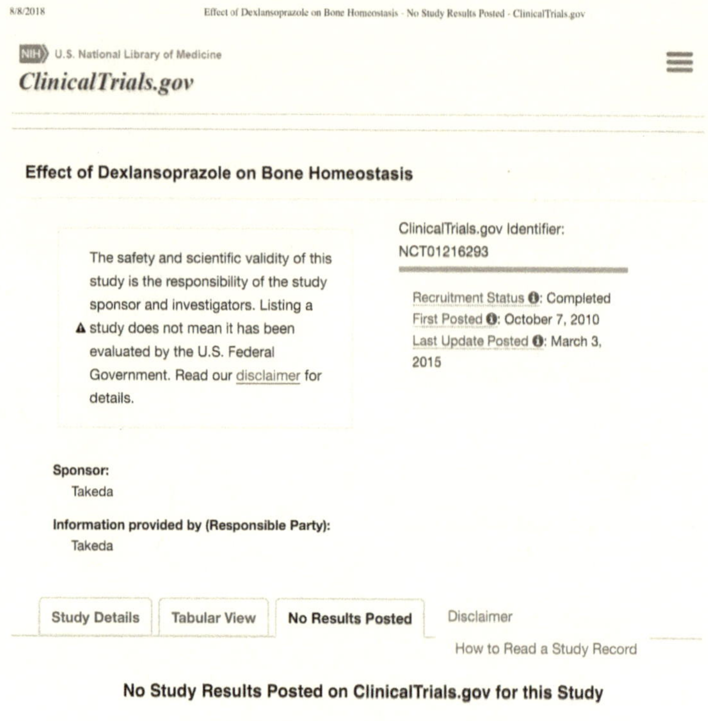

Recruitment Status ❶:	Completed
Actual Primary Completion Date ❶:	August 2014
Actual Study Completion Date ❶:	February 2015

WITH THE IMPORTANCE given to this topic why has it slipped through the cracks? There is "No Results Posted" for this study. What does that mean?

. . .

PHARMACEUTICAL COMPANIES ARE ONLY ALLOWED to promote what has been approved by the Federal Drug Administration and is in the product label. There should be a product information sheet with every prescription a patient receives, however they are rarely looked at.

According to an article by Dr. Amnon Sonnenberg in the *Yale Journal of Biology and Medicine*, "Clinical Epidemiology and Natural History of Gastroesophageal Reflux Disease"[4], looking at the patients "with GERD symptoms, about 20 percent are found to have erosive esophagitis, while ulcers or strictures are found in less than 5 percent of all patients with erosive esophagitis." What this information means, is that since only 20 percent of GERD patients have erosive esophagitis, the Dexilant 60mg sales data should be in that same 20 percent range, leaving Dexilant 30mg sales data at around 80 percent. The fact that 60mg sales are over 90 percent shows that it is due to the promotion and sampling of only that 60mg dose.

THE DEXILANT PACKAGE INSERT has several important things to notice:

The only three FDA approved indications:

-30mg for Maintenance of Healed EE and Relief of Heartburn. Controlled studies did not extend beyond 6 months.

-30mg for Symptomatic Non-Erosive GERD for 4 weeks.

-60mg for Healing of EE for 8 weeks.

THE "WARNINGS AND PRECAUTIONS" section of the package insert is to make peartbents and physicians aware of potential issues. The main one this book is about is Bone Fractures but the Dexilant "Warnings and Precautions" are:

Gastric Malignancy

Acute Interstitial Nephritis
Clostridium difficile-Associated Diarrhea
Bone Fracture
Cutaneous and Systemic Lupus Erythematosus
Cyanocobalamin (Vitamin B12) Deficiency
Hypomagnesemia
Interactions with Investigations for Neuroendocrine Tumors
Interaction with Methotrexate
Fundic Gland Polyps

5.4 Bone Fracture

Several published observational studies suggest that PPI therapy may be associated with an increased risk for osteoporosis-related fractures of the hip, wrist or spine. The risk of fracture was increased in patients who received high-dose, defined as multiple daily doses, and long-term PPI therapy (a year or longer). Patients should use the lowest dose and shortest duration of PPI therapy appropriate to the conditions being treated. Patients at risk for osteoporosis-related fractures should be managed according to established treatment guidelines [see Dosage and Administration (2), Adverse Reactions (6.2)].

14.2 MAINTENANCE of Healed Erosive Esophagitis and Relief of Heartburn in Adults

A multi-center, double-blind, placebo-controlled, randomized study was conducted in patients who successfully completed an EE study and showed endoscopically confirmed healed EE. Maintenance of healing and symptom resolution over a six month period was evaluated with DEXILANT 30 or 60 mg once daily compared to placebo. A total of 445 patients were enrolled and ranged in age from 18 to 85 years (median age 49 years), with

52% female. Race was distributed as follows: 90% Caucasian, 5% Black and 5% Other.

Sixty six percent of patients treated with 30 mg of DEXILANT remained healed over the six month time period as confirmed by endoscopy (see Table 9).

DEXILANT 60 mg once daily was studied and did not provide additional clinical benefit over DEXILANT 30 mg once daily.

HEARTBURN IS the main reason for which PPI's are prescribed. If the package insert states that 60mg did not provide additional clinical benefit over 30mg, why is 60mg the preferred dose?

An important thing to consider is, how is erosive esophagitis (EE) diagnosed? EE is only diagnosed through an endoscopy, which is a visual examination of the esophagus by using a scope. Unless in an extreme circumstance, primary care providers are not diagnosing EE since they don't have the equipment or the expertise to do so. Since primary care providers are not diagnosing EE, they should not be prescribing Dexilant 60mg. If they were going to put a patient on Dexilant, it should be at the 30mg dose.

The tricky situation, is that there is nothing illegal with the primary care provider writing a 60mg prescription for any reason they see fit. The provider went to medical school and acquired the proper training necessary to treat and prescribe medication for their patients. The issue is whether the pharmaceutical company influenced them to write the prescription for an off-label use.

The FDA approved indication for 60mg of Dexilant is for EE. Since EE can only be diagnosed through visual confirmation why are the primary care providers starting at 60mg? Is it because the representatives only sample and talk about 60mg?

Takeda Pharmaceuticals' defense, from court documents, is

that if anything negative occurs from the physician writing Dexilant 60mg, it is the fault of the physician. Regardless of what the
pharmaceutical representatives say, and what samples are
present in the sample closet, it is the responsibility of the physician to have read the Package Insert and to know what the correct
dose is.

In my case we provided several sources showing that physicians do not read package inserts:

C. Physicians Are Often Unaware of the Indications for the
Prescriptions They Write and Do Not Generally Read Drug
Labels ("Package Inserts")

252. Physicians generally do not have the time to read the
labels for the drugs they prescribe and rely on pharmaceutical
sales representatives to provide information to them regarding
the drugs they promote that is accurate and not misleading.

253. In a national survey conducted by physicians from the
University of Virginia and the University of Chicago and
published in the Journal of Pharmacoepidemiology and Drug
Safety in 2009 (the "Indication Study")[5], the researchers surveyed
1199 physicians regarding their knowledge of FDA approved indications of medications (i.e. physicians were asked "Is this an FDA-
approved indication [for a specific drug]?" With the answer
options "Yes," "No" and "Don't Know."

254. Although 79% of the physicians reported that the importance of FDA labeling as a general factor guiding their
prescribing was either "very important" or "somewhat important," the data showed that the average respondent accurately
identified the FDA-approval status in only 55% of the drug indications queried. Moreover, the accuracy of primary care physicians
was even lower – with only 42% of such physicians responding
correctly regarding drug indications.

255. The authors of the Indication Study concluded that:

"a significant minority of physicians also prescribe some drugs for off-label indications, in the belief that they are approved for such uses, despite uncertain or no supporting evidence. These results indicate an urgent need for effective methods of disseminating information to physicians about the level of evidence supporting off-label drug uses, with specific attention to common off-label uses known to be ineffective or to carry unacceptable risk of harm."

256. Indeed, a 2006 study published by the American Medical Association in the Annals of Internal Medicine concluded that almost three quarters (73%) of off-label prescriptions are written for conditions "for which there is little or no scientific support for efficacy."[6]

257. The fact that physicians are frequently unaware of prescription drug indications is not surprising in light of data that the vast majority of physicians do not read drug labels. The New York Times reported in 2006 that "fewer than one in 10 physicians routinely read drug labels."[7]

258. More recently, Dr. Califf, a practicing cardiologist and Professor of Cardiology at Duke University and the Vice Chancellor for Clinical Research and Director of the Duke Translational Medicine Institute, stated in a 2009 interview that "less than 1 percent of physicians have seen a label in the last year." (emphasis added).[8]

259. Further, as stated in an article in the Journal of the American Medical Association, physicians who must "evaluate, diagnose, and initiate treatment for a patient within the limits of a 12-minute office visit have inadequate time to effectively counsel patients about their medications." Indeed, Dr. Janet Woodcock, the director of the Center for Drug Evaluation and Research (CDER), the division of the FDA responsible for approving new drugs and ensuring the safety and effectiveness of all drugs, has publicly stated her concern about physicians review of drug labels indicating

that doctors have only "30 seconds to make that prescribing decision."[9]

260. Further supporting this conclusion – even by high-level officials in the FDA – Dr. William Hubbard, a former FDA associate commissioner stated in an August 2008 journal article that "I think the FDA would love for doctors to read the package inserts . . . but they don't."[10]

261. And another former FDA associate commissioner, Peter Pitts states that "for better or worse, doctors don't have the time to sit down and carefully read medical articles discussing off-label use, or even physician package inserts."[11]

ACCORDING TO THE DEXILANT.COM WEBSITE, patients can use coupon cards for 30 and 90-day prescriptions. An important note about the 90-day promotion, it doesn't say anything about 30mg even though only the 30mg is indicated for anything more than 8 weeks.

The Dexilant patent expires in 2020, and Par Pharmaceuticals already has FDA approval to make the first generic version of dexlansoprazole. An interesting fact is that Par Pharmaceuticals is only going to make 60mg. Why would they only produce a 60mg dose when GERD, which is only indicated for the 30mg, is the predominant diagnosis for patients taking PPI's? I would guess that it is because Takeda created the market demand for 60mg. Even though 60 mg of dexlansoprazole is double the FDA indicated dose for GERD, and dexlansoprazole includes an FDA warning about using the lowest dose for the shortest duration, only the 60 mg generic is set to be made.

<u>DEXILANT MEDICATION GUIDE,</u> produced by Takeda Pharmaceuticals.

DEXILANT (decks-i-launt) (dexlansoprazole) delayed-release capsules, for oral use

Read this Medication Guide before you start taking DEXILANT and each time you get a refill. There may be new information. This information does not take the place of talking to your doctor about your medical condition or your treatment.

What is the most important information that I should know about DEXILANT?

DEXILANT may help your acid-related symptoms, but you could still have serious stomach problems. Talk with your doctor.

DEXILANT can cause serious side effects, including:

• **A type of kidney problem (acute interstitial nephritis).** Some people who take proton pump inhibitor (PPI) medicines, including DEXILANT, may develop a kidney problem called acute interstitial nephritis, that can happen at any time during treatment with PPI medicines. Call your doctor right away if you have a decrease in the amount that you urinate or if you have blood in your urine.

• **Diarrhea.** DEXILANT may increase your risk of getting severe diarrhea. This diarrhea may be caused by an infection (Clostridium difficile) in your intestines. Call your doctor right away if you have watery stool, stomach pain, and fever that does not go away.

• **Bone fractures.** People who take multiple daily doses of PPI medicines for a long period of time (a year or longer) may have an increased risk of fractures of the hip, wrist or spine. You should take DEXILANT exactly as prescribed, at the lowest dose possible for your treatment and for the shortest time needed. Talk to your doctor about your risk of bone fracture if you take DEXILANT.

• **Certain types of lupus erythematosus.** Lupus erythematosus is an autoimmune disorder (the body's immune cells attack other cells or organs in the body). Some people who take PPI medicines may develop certain types of lupus erythematosus or have worsening of the lupus they already have. Call your doctor right away if you have new or worsening joint pain or a rash on your cheeks or arms that gets worse in the sun. DEXILANT can have other serious side effects. See "**What are the possible side effects of DEXILANT?**"

9

DEXILANT AND BONE FRACTURES

A search for "PPI's and bone fractures" will reveal countless articles and studies on the topic. One thing they have in common is that patients should use the lowest dose for the shortest duration of time. There aren't any published studies on Dexilant and broken bones data specifically. Despite the required study by Takeda, no results have been posted by the FDA, which is curious given that the required deadline was years ago. Since the data hasn't been collected, I will be seeking independent data on my website: www.appleQD.com. It is reasonable that people experienced broken bones but have not attributed it to taking high doses of Dexilant. Using the amount of literature on high dose PPI's, along with the FDA concerns, and the millions of Dexilant prescriptions filled, it should be enough to encourage further investigation. The medical literature shows that bones can become brittle during long-term use of high dose PPI's. If you have experienced a broken bone while on Dexilant 60mg I would encourage you to inform your physician and also go to my website, www.appleQD.com, to add yourself to the list. The information you should provide is:

-Your name and contact information including email address
-Dates you took Dexilant
-Dosage strength of Dexilant
-Date and bone broken

THE FOLLOWING ARE two Safety Announcements from the FDA.

Safety Announcement[1]:

[05-25-2010] The U.S. Food and Drug Administration (FDA) is revising the prescription and over-the-counter (OTC) labels for a class of drugs called proton pump inhibitors to include new safety information about a possible increased risk of fractures of the hip, wrist, and spine with the use of these medications.

Proton pump inhibitors work by reducing the amount of acid in the stomach. Nexium, Dexilant, Prilosec, Zegerid, Prevacid, Protonix, Aciphex, and Vimovo are available by prescription to treat conditions such as gastroesophageal reflux disease (GERD), stomach and small intestine ulcers, and inflammation of the esophagus. Prilosec OTC, Zegerid OTC, and Prevacid 24HR are sold over-the-counter (OTC) for the treatment of frequent heartburn.

The new safety information is based on FDA's review of several epidemiological studies that reported an increased risk of fractures of the hip, wrist, and spine with proton pump inhibitor use. Some studies found that those at greatest risk for these fractures received high doses of proton pump inhibitors or used them for one year or more (see Data Summary section). The majority of the studies evaluated individuals 50 years of age or older and the increased risk of fracture primarily was observed in this age group.

While the greatest increased risk for fractures in these studies involved people who had been taking prescription proton pump inhibitors for at least one year or who had been taking high doses of the prescription medications (not available over-the-counter), as a precaution, the "Drug Facts" label on the OTC proton pump inhibitors (indicated for 14 days of continuous use) also is being revised to include information about this risk.

Healthcare professionals and users of proton pump inhibitors should be aware of the possible increased risk of fractures of the hip, wrist, and spine with the use of proton pump inhibitors, and weigh the known benefits against the potential risks when deciding to use them.

Additional Information for Healthcare Professionals

• Proton pump inhibitors provide important benefits for many patients in treating or preventing conditions such as erosive esophagitis, nonsteroidal anti-inflammatory drug-induced ulcers and gastroesophageal reflux disease.

• Be aware of the increased risk of fractures of the hip, wrist, and spine seen in some observational studies in patients using proton pump inhibitors.

• When prescribing proton pump inhibitors, consider whether a lower dose or shorter duration of therapy would adequately treat the patient's condition.

• Follow the recommendations in the product labeling when prescribing proton pump inhibitors.

• Individuals at risk for osteoporosis should have their bone status managed according to current clinical practice, and should take adequate vitamin D and calcium supplementation.

• Report any adverse events with proton pump inhibitors to FDA's MedWatch program using the information at the bottom of the page in the "Contact Us" box.

UPDATE: 3/23/2011

FDA has determined an osteoporosis and fracture warning on the over-the-counter (OTC) proton pump inhibitor (PPI) medication "Drug Facts" label is not indicated at this time. Following a thorough review of available safety data, FDA has concluded that fracture risk with short-term, low dose PPI use is unlikely.

The available data show that patients at highest risk for fractures received high doses of prescription PPIs (higher than OTC PPI doses) and/or used a PPI for one year or more.

In contrast to prescription PPIs, OTC PPIs are marketed at low doses and are only intended for a 14 day course of treatment up to 3 times per year. FDA acknowledges that consumers, either on their own, or based on a healthcare professional's recommendation, may take these products for periods of time that exceed the directions on the OTC label. Healthcare professionals should be aware of the risk for fracture if they are recommending use of OTC PPIs at higher doses or for longer periods of time than in the OTC PPI label.

To hit the main points of those two FDA Safety Announcements, taking a high dose PPI can cause bone fractures whereas taking a low dose PPI for a short duration is thought to be safe (as of 3/23/2011).

Even with this information, Takeda continued to promote Dexilant at 60mg for GERD, which is double the indicated dose according to the FDA approved package insert. The FDA approved package insert also has the statement that "Dexilant 60mg was studied and did not provide additional clinical benefit over Dexilant 30mg once daily" regarding GERD.

A 2006 article in the *Journal of the American Medical Association (JAMA)*, "Long-term Proton Pump Inhibitor Therapy and Risk of Hip Fracture"[2], a team lead by study author Dr. Yu-Xiao Yang collected statistics on 13,556 people with hip fractures and 135,386 healthy people, all aged 50 or older. The researchers discovered that taking a proton pump inhibitor for more than one year increased the threat of hip fracture by 44%, compared with people not taking PPI's. Additionally, the risk was 2.6 times higher among people who took high doses over a long period. Yang's team found the risk of hip fracture increased with both the dosage and the duration of proton pump inhibitor therapy. The team also noted that, "the mortality rate during the first year after a hip fracture is 20%. Among those who survived this period, 1 in 5 requires nursing home care." The concern with PPI's and bone fractures, according to Dr. Yang et al, has to do with, "PPI's may interfere with calcium absorption through induction of hypochlorhydria but they also may reduce bone resorption through inhibition of osteoclastic vacuolar proton pumps."

Dr. Liwei Wang et al wrote an article published in 2017 in *Nature,* "Proton Pump Inhibitors and the Risk for Fracture at Specific Sites: Data Mining of the FDA Adverse Event Reporting System"[3]. Dr. Wang et al expanded the scope of bone fractures to the entire body and showed the increasing trend of PPI related fractures from 2004 – 2011.

A 2011 article published in *The American Journal of Medicine,* "Proton Pump Inhibitors and Risk of Fractures: a Meta-analysis of 11 International Studies"[4] Dr. Yu et al aims to provide more information to the debate. They concluded, "In this meta-analysis of observational studies, PPIs modestly increased the risk of hip, spine, and any-site fractures, whereas H2RAs were not associated with fracture risk."

According to Vaezi et al in the journal *Gastroenterology* 2017;153:35-48, "Complications of Proton Pump Inhibitor Therapy"[5], the issue with bone fractures and osteoporosis, as related to PPI use, involves the reduction of gastric acidity with subsequent hypergastrinemia. (In plain English, gastric acidity refers to how PPI's reduce heartburn by lowering the amount of acid in the stomach by shutting down the parietal cells. Hypergastrinemia is defined as the presence of excess gastrin in the blood.)

The reduction of gastric acidity may lead to malabsorption of calcium and vitamin B12. Vitamin B12 deficiency may lead to homocysteinemia linked to reduced bone strength. Hypergastrinemia may lead to secondary hyperparathyroidism.

In a new study published in 2018 by *The Journal of Clinical Endocrinology & Metabolism* titled, "Fractures Tied to Increased Risk of Death for up to 10 Years"[6] shows that people over the age of 50 can have up to a 25 percent mortality risk after a broken bone. The researchers looked at 21,000 women and 9,500 men over the age of 50 who have experienced a fracture in 2001. They were followed for the next 10 years and compared to people without fractures. After the 10 years, 10,668 of the women and 4,745 of the men had died. After adjusting for the average mortality rates from other causes, it was determined that there is an "excess mortality risk linked to having had a fracture."

THE DEXILANT PACKAGE Insert dated June 2018 states:

5.4 Bone Fracture

Several published observational studies suggest that PPI therapy may be associated with an increased risk for osteoporosis-related fractures of the hip, wrist or spine. The risk of fracture was increased in patients who received high-dose, defined as multiple daily doses, and long-term PPI therapy (a year or longer). Patients should use the lowest dose and shortest duration of PPI therapy appropriate to the conditions being treated. Patients at risk for osteoporosis-related fractures should be managed according to established treatment guidelines [see Dosage and Administration (2), Adverse Reactions (6.2)].

THE IMPORTANT THINGS TO note in the Bone Fracture section are:

"The risk of fracture was increased in patients who received high-dose, defined as multiple daily doses, and long term PPI therapy."

DEXILANT 60MG IS ONLY INDICATED for erosive esophagitis for 8 weeks and the 30mg dose should be the most common for GERD. Patients taking 60mg, without ever trying 30mg, are taking high-dose. Dexilant is a PPI with a Dual Delayed Release, which means multiple doses are released from the same capsule. So, patients are receiving both a high dose and multiple doses at the same time with Dexilant 60mg.

"PATIENTS SHOULD USE the lowest dose and shortest duration of PPI therapy."

GERD is a common condition with approximately 20 percent of the adult U.S. population effected weekly, according to Dr. S.D. Martinez *et al.* in a 2003 article, "Non-erosive reflex disease (NERD) - acid reflux and symptom patterns"[7] from *Alimentary Pharmacology & Therapeutics*. The article explains that erosive esophagitis is not as common effecting only approximately 6 percent of the adult U.S. population (30 percent of the 20 percent). With erosive esophagitis in such a low percentage of patients, why is the 60mg dose of Dexilant used so much?

TAP PHARMACEUTICALS SUBMITTED its New Drug Application (NDA) for Kapidex in December 2007. In its NDA, TAP sought approval of 30, 60 and 90 mg dosages of Kapidex. The FDA approved 60mg for healing erosive esophagitis for 8 weeks, 30mg for maintaining healed erosive esophagitis, and 30mg for GERD.

There were multiple doctors at the FDA working on the NDA for Kapidex, two of the main researchers were Dr. Keith B. St.

Amand and Dr. Tamara Johnson. In Dr. St. Amand's summary, as noted on the FDA website concerning the Risk/Benefit Assessment:[8]

"SINCE THIS REVIEW evaluated only the efficacy of the product, it is difficult to provide a detailed risk/benefit assessment here. However, the reviewer is aware of several safety concerns that have arisen with this application (see Dr. Tamera Johnson's review of safety). Although dexlansoprazole is effective for all 3 indications being sought, the reviewer strongly believes that no convincing evidence of additional benefit over existing therapies has been demonstrated in the current application.

Due to this lack of additional benefit along with the safety concerns that have been voiced in Dr. Johnson's review, the reviewer believes that the benefit/risk profile for dexlansoprazole is unfavorable at this time, and that future studies should be required to clarify the nature of the potential safety signal before any approval for marketing is granted."[9]

DR. TAMARA JOHNSON's RISK/BENEFIT Assessment shows concern for both safety and "benefit over the 5 currently marketed PPI's":

"DEXLANSOPRAZOLE BELONGS to the drug class of proton pump inhibitors (PPI); a class which now houses 5 marketed products (see section 2.2.) Throughout its Phase 3 development program, dexlansoprazole has demonstrated greater benefit for the symptomatic GERD and the erosive esophagitis patient populations when compared to placebo and lansoprazole (Prevacid) 30mg. Although, as discussed in the efficacy review by Dr. St. Amand, dexlansoprazole provides no additional benefit over the 5 currently marketed PPI's, the benefit of dexlansoprazole outweighs the risk of adverse events. Safety concern about a potentially increased risk of ischemic cardiovascular adverse events among dexlansoprazole 30mg subjects was diminished due to previous cardiac medical history in the subjects and absence of similarly increased risk among dexlansoprazole 60mg and 90mg treatment groups. Labeling recommendations have been advised to address this potential concern. This reviewer, however, remains with concern for fracture/injury-related adverse events, which occurred at greater incidence with dexlansoprazole than its comparators. (See section 7 Safety Summary) In order to manage this potential risk, a post-marketing study and labeling recommendations are advised."[10]

DUE TO THE concern of bone fractures, Kapidex was required to conduct a post-marketing clinical trial by the FDA as part of their approval process. The following is from the FDA:[11]

TAKEDA WILL CONDUCT a clinical trial to evaluate the effect of Kapidex (dexlansoprazole) Delayed Release Capsules on bone homeostasis. The primary endpoint will be biomarkers of bone formation and bone resorption. Treatments will include: placebo, dexlansoprazole and esomeprazole (Nexium).

The timetable you submitted on January 12, 2009, states that you will conduct this trial according to the following timetable:

FINAL PROTOCOL SUBMISSION: August 31, 2009
    Trial Start Date:October 31, 2009
    Final Report Submission: December 31, 2011

· · ·

*As of the writing this book in November 2018 the results of the clinical trial have not been released and the FDA website shows "No Results Posted".[12]

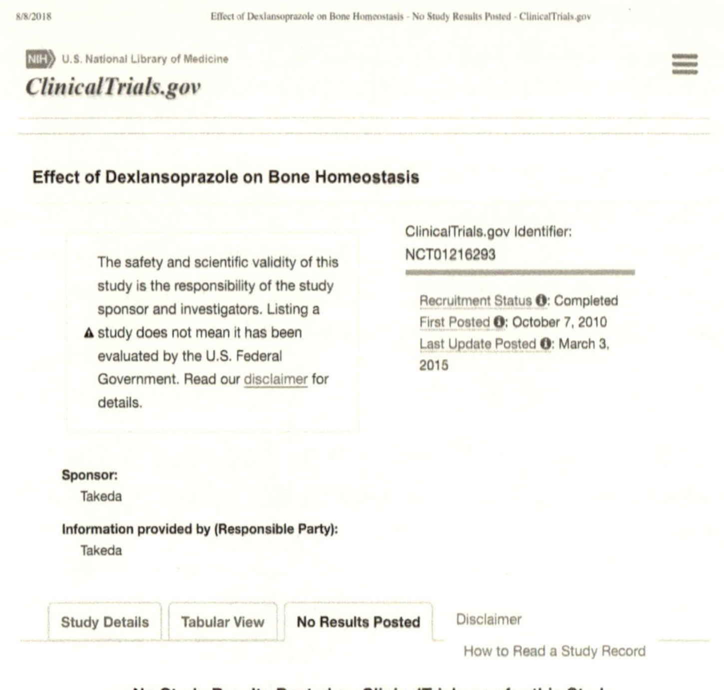

Recruitment Status :	Completed
Actual Primary Completion Date :	August 2014
Actual Study Completion Date :	February 2015

10

TATUM V. TAKEDA PHARMACEUTICALS

According to Drugwatch.com[1], Takeda reached a settlement on a case involving a Prevacid bone fracture lawsuit in 2014. The amount of the settlement and the specifics were not available.

David S. Tatum alleges that Prevacid, which was designed, manufactured, and marketed by Takeda, weakened his bones, ultimately leading to his hip fractures. His case began in 2012 in the Eastern District of Pennsylvania, *David S. Tatum v. Takeda Pharmaceuticals.*[2]

Mr. Tatum was prescribed, and used Prevacid from May 2006 through May 2010. In May 2010 he experienced severe hip pain which was determined to be Stage 3 Avascular Necrosis of the left hip. He was forced to undergo a total hip replacement from the injury. Mr. Tatum claims that his injury was the result of his use of Prevacid, causing his bones to become weakened and brittle. He also claims that Takeda Pharmaceuticals was aware of, and concealed the bone fracture risk.

Takeda filed motions in an attempt to dismiss the case, which ended up before Judge Jan Dubois of the Eastern District of Pennsylvania. On October 19, 2012, Judge Dubois split her decision allowing some of the claims to be dismissed but allowing the case to move forward.

The following are documents from the case, however, I could not find any court documentation after Judge Dubois' order allowing the case to proceed. I believe that the Prevacid bone fracture settlement in 2014, as reported by Drugwatch, was Mr. Tatum's case.

Judge Dubois concluded that the following sections of the case may proceed:

Count V – negligent misrepresentation

Count VI – breach of express warranty

Count VII – breach of implied warranty for a particular purpose

Count VIII – breach of implied warranty of merchantability

Count X – strict product liability: manufacturing defect

Count XII – fraudulent concealment

Count XIV – violations of Pennsylvania Unfair Trade Practices and Consumer Protection Law

IN HER DECISION, Judge Dubois writes:

"Tatum alleges that defendants falsely represented "that PREVACID was safe and fit for its intended purpose, was of merchantable quality, did not produce any dangerous side effects, and had been adequately tested." This is a sufficiently specific allegation. Thus, the motion to dismiss with respect to the claim for negligent misrepresentation asserted in Count V is denied."

THE TATUM CASE is concerned with the drug Prevacid. Prevacid is made by Takeda Pharmaceuticals and its generic name is lansoprazole. Dexilant is also made by Takeda Pharmaceuticals and its generic name is dexlansoprazole. Dexilant is the R-enantiomer of Prevacid and in the FDA approved product information, it states that it was initially approved in 1995 as lansoprazole.

. . .

THIS IS **the edited version of the document to make it easier to read for the non-lawyer. The original unedited version is at the end of the chapter.**

IN THE UNITED STATES DISTRICT COURT FOR THE EASTERN DISTRICT OF PENNSYLVANIA

_________________________________ DAVID S. TATUM, :

Plaintiff, v.
TAKEDA   PHARMACEUTICALS,   Defendant.

____

DuBois, J.
I. INTRODUCTION
CIVIL ACTION NO. 12-1114

MEMORANDUM

October 18, 2012

This is a product liability action in which plaintiff David S. Tatum alleges that the PREVACID designed, manufactured, and marketed by defendants weakened his bones, ultimately leading to hip fractures. The defendants filed a motion to dismiss many of the claims in Tatum's First Amended Complaint. For the reasons that follow, the Court grants in part and denies in part defendants' motion.

II. BACKGROUND

Tatum was prescribed PREVACID, a pharmaceutical drug designed, manufactured, and marketed by defendants. After taking PREVACID, Tatum began feeling pain in his left hip, and he was later diagnosed with Stage III Avascular Necrosis. Tatum's bones became weakened or brittle, causing multiple fractures. As a result, he underwent total hip replacement surgery.

Tatum claims that defendants were aware of the risks of PREVACID, but chose not to disclose them. His First Amended Complaint contains fourteen counts: Count I – equitable tolling of applicable statute of limitations; Count II – negligence; Count III – negligent failure to adequately warn; Count IV – negligence per se; Count V – negligent misrepresentation; Count VI – breach of express warranty; Count VII – breach of implied warranty for a particular purpose; Count VIII – breach of implied warranty of merchantability; Count IX – strict product liability: defective design; Count X – strict product liability: manufacturing defect; Count XI – strict product liability: failure to warn; Count XII – fraudulent concealment; Count XIII – unjust enrichment; and Count XIV – violations of Pennsylvania Unfair Trade Practices and Consumer Protection Law. Tatum additionally alleges that he is entitled to punitive damages.

Defendants have moved to dismiss Count I, Counts V to XIV, and the request for punitive damages.

III. STANDARD OF REVIEW

To survive a motion to dismiss under Rule 12(b)(6), a civil plaintiff must allege facts that "'raise a right to relief above the speculative level.'" A complaint must contain "sufficient factual matter, accepted as true, to 'state a claim to relief that is plausible on its face.'" "The tenet that a court must accept as true all of the allegations contained in a complaint is inapplicable to legal conclusions. Threadbare recitals of the elements of a cause of action, supported by mere conclusory statements, do not suffice."

IV . DISCUSSION

Defendants have moved to dismiss eleven of the fourteen counts in the First Amended Complaint, in addition to Tatum's request for punitive damages. The Court will address each in turn.

A. Count I: Equitable Tolling

Defendants initially move to dismiss Tatum's claim for equitable tolling alleged in Count I. Tatum alleges that "the running of any statute of limitations has been tolled by reason of Defendants' fraudulent concealment." Fraudulent concealment is a doctrine which "serves to toll the running of the statute of limitations." Unlike the tort of fraudulent concealment alleged in Count XII, this doctrine is not an independent cause of action. Thus, Count I is dismissed with prejudice.

It appears that by moving to dismiss Count I, defendants are also attempting to attack Tatum's tort claims, which are subject to a two-year statute of limitations. Generally, "a limitations defense must be raised in the answer, since Rule 12(b) does not permit it to be raised by motion." However, the "Third Circuit Rule" allows defendants to raise a limitations defense in a Rule 12(b)(6) motion where the "time alleged in the statement of a claim shows that the cause of action has not been brought within the statute of limitations."

Tatum filed his initial Complaint on March 1, 2012. In his First Amended Complaint, he states that "at no point prior to March 2010 had Plaintiff experienced any type of abnormal hip pain . . . ." As this allegation falls within the two-year period, the Court will not dismiss any claims on statute of limitations grounds on the present state of the record.

B. Counts IX, X, and XI: Strict Liability Claims

The Court next addresses Tatum's strict liability claims. Counts IX and XI which assert claims for strict liability based on design defect and strict liability based on failure to warn are not permitted under Pennsylvania law. Applying comment k to 402A of the Restatement (Second) of Torts, the Pennsylvania Supreme Court ruled that "where the adequacy of warnings associated with prescription drugs is at issue, the failure of the manufacturer to exercise reasonable care to warn of dangers, i.e., the manufacturer's negligence, is the only recognized basis of liability." As a result, Tatum cannot bring strict liability claims for design defect or failure to warn.

Count X which alleges a claim of strict liability based on

manufacturing defect, however, is permissible. Many courts have interpreted Hahn broadly to preclude all strict liability claims. However, this Court agrees with the decision in Doughtery, where the court concluded that strict liability claims for manufacturing defects are not prohibited.

Tatum's claims in Count IX for strict liability based on design defect and Count XI for strict liability based on failure to warn are dismissed with prejudice. The strict liability claim based on manufacturing defect asserted in Count X is permitted under Pennsylvania Law. Thus, the motion to dismiss with respect to the claim for strict liability based on manufacturing defect asserted in Count X is denied.

C. Counts VI, VII, and VIII: Breach of Warranty Claims

Defendants further move to dismiss Tatum's breach of warranty claims. In his First Amended Complaint, Tatum alleges breach of implied warranty of merchantability in Count VIII, breach of implied warranty for a particular purpose in Count VII, and breach of express warranty in Count VI.

(a) Counts VII and VIII: Breach of Implied Warranty of Fitness for a Particular Purpose and Breach of Implied Warranty of Merchantability

"The theories of strict liability and breach of the implied warranty of merchantability are parallel theories of recovery, one in contract and the other in tort." As discussed above, strict liability claims based on design defect or failure to warn are not permissible in Pennsylvania. "It would thus be inconsistent to exempt a manufacturer . . . from strict liability under comment k and apply a negligence standard to determine liability for a design defect or a failure to warn, but allow a plaintiff to recover for the same alleged defect under a theory of breach of the implied warranty of merchantability." The same analysis applies to the implied warranty of fitness for a particular purpose. Both claims are not cognizable under Pennsylvania law to the extent they are based on a design defect or failure to warn, but are permissible if based on manufacturing defect or any other theory. Thus, the motion to dismiss with respect to the claims, as limited by this Memorandum, for breach of the implied warranty fitness for a particular purpose asserted in Count VII and for breach of the implied warranty of merchantability asserted in Count VIII is denied.

(b) Count VI: Breach of Express Warranty

Tatum's remaining breach of warranty claim is for breach of express warranty. Federal courts are split concerning whether an express warranty claim against prescription drug manufacturers is permissible under Pennsylvania law. This Court concludes that such a claim is permitted. "While the reasoning of comment k may prevent certain warranties or promises from being implied by law," that is not a "basis for declining to enforce a contractual promise expressly and voluntarily made by a manufacturer of prescription drugs or devices." Thus, the motion to dismiss with respect to the claim for breach of an express warranty asserted in Count VI is denied.

D. Count V: Negligent Misrepresentation

Defendants additionally move to dismiss Tatum's claim for negligent misrepresentation alleged in Count V because Tatum failed to allege his claim with the particularity required by Federal Rule of Civil Procedure 9(b). Although a plaintiff must plead negligent misrepresentation with a degree of specificity, Rule 9(b) does not govern negligent misrepresentation claims. Tatum alleges that defendants falsely represented "that PREVACID was safe and fit for its intended purpose, was of merchantable quality, did not produce any dangerous side effects, and had been adequately tested." This is a sufficiently specific allegation. Thus, the motion to dismiss with respect to the claim for negligent misrepresentation asserted in Count V is denied.

E. Counts XII and XIV: Fraudulent Concealment and Violations of Pennsylvania's Unfair Trade Practices and Consumer Protection Law

Defendants next move to dismiss Tatum's claims for fraudulent concealment alleged in Count XII and for violations of Pennsylvania's Unfair Trade Practices and Consumer Protection Law, alleged in Count XIV. Fraudulent concealment "has the same elements as intentional misrepresentation except in the case of intentional non-disclosure, the party intentionally conceals a material fact rather than making an affirmative misrepresentation."

Section 201-3 of the UTPCPL makes "unfair methods of competition and unfair or deceptive acts or practices in the conduct of any trade or commerce . . . unlawful." Section 201-2(4), the so- called "catch-all" definition, defines "unfair methods of competition and unfair or deceptive acts or practices" as "engaging in any other fraudulent or deceptive conduct which creates a likelihood of confusion or of misunderstanding." "A plaintiff may succeed under the catch-all provision by satisfying the elements of common-law fraud." The fraud can be based on the intentional concealment of information. Thus, Tatum's claims for fraudulent concealment and for violations of the UTPCPL overlap.

Defendants argue that both claims, which are based on intentional conduct, should be dismissed because they "do not rest on a theory of negligence." For this proposition, defendants cite the Pennsylvania Supreme Court's statement in Hahn that "where the adequacy of warnings associated with prescription drugs is at issue, the failure of the manufacturer to exercise reasonable care to warn of dangers, i.e., the manufacturer's negligence, is the only recognized basis of liability."

This Court disagrees. The court in Hahn stated that a seller of prescription drugs must not only warn of risks of which he reasonably should have knowledge, but also warn of risks of which he did, in fact, have knowledge. Accordingly, Hahn does not preclude claims where the plaintiff alleges that the seller had knowledge of the risks of prescription drugs and intentionally concealed them.

For this reason, the motion to dismiss with respect to the claims for fraudulent concealment asserted in Count XII and for violations of Pennsylvania's Unfair Trade Practices and Consumer Protection Law asserted in Count XIV is denied. Since Tatum has stated a claim under the "fraud prong" of the catch- all provision of the UTPCPL, the Court does not address the "deceptive conduct" prong of the catch-all provision or the other provisions of the UPTCPL referenced in the First Amended Complaint.

F. Count XIII: Unjust Enrichment

Defendants also move to dismiss Tatum's claim for unjust enrichment alleged in Count XIII. "Under Pennsylvania law, the plaintiff must demonstrate that he conferred a benefit on the defendant, that the defendant knew of the benefit and accepted or retained it, and that it would be inequitable to allow the defendant to keep the benefit without paying for it." However, "unjust enrichment is not a substitute for failed tort claims in Pennsylvania . . . ."

This is not a case in which a claim for unjust enrichment is appropriate. Specifically, there is no allegation that defendants refused to provide a service or goods after Tatum provided defendants with a benefit. Thus, Tatum's claim in Count XIII for unjust enrichment is dismissed with prejudice.

G. Punitive Damages

Finally, defendants move to dismiss Tatum's request for punitive damages. Defendants argue that under Pennsylvania law, punitive damages are not an independent cause of action. That is correct. However, Tatum did not assert an independent claim for punitive damages in the First Amended Complaint. Rather, he requested punitive damages as a remedy. Punitive damages are properly alleged in the First Amended Complaint.

V . CONCLUSION

For the reasons set forth above, the Court grants in part and denies in part defendants' motion to dismiss. Count I – equitable tolling of applicable statute of limitations; Count IX – strict product liability: defective design; Count XI – strict product liability: failure to warn; and Count XIII – unjust enrichment; are dismissed with prejudice.

The claims remaining for adjudication are: Count V – negligent misrepresentation; Count VI – breach of express warranty; Count VII – breach of implied warranty for a particular purpose; Count VIII – breach of implied warranty of merchantability; Count X – strict product liability: manufacturing defect; Count XII – fraudulent concealment; and Count XIV – violations of Pennsylvania Unfair Trade Practices and Consumer Protection Law.

The Court concludes that many of Tatum's remaining claims are redundant or otherwise unnecessary, making this case unduly complicated. At the preliminary pretrial conference, the Court will address narrowing the scope of the issues presented.

An appropriate order follows.

United States District Court,

E.D. Pennsylvania.

David S. TATUM, Plaintiff,

v.

TAKEDA PHARMACEUTICALS NORTH AMERICA, INC.

Civil Action No. 12–1114.

Oct. 19, 2012.

Attorneys and Law Firms

Claudine Q. Homolash, Sheller P.C., Philadelphia, PA, Kenneth G. Gilman, Gilman Law LLP, Bonita Springs, FL, for Plaintiff.

Tiffany M. Alexander, Campbell Campbell Edwards & Conroy, Wayne, PA, for Defendants.

. . .

ORDER

JAN E. DuBOIS, District Judge.

AND NOW, this 18th day of October, 2012, upon consideration of Defendants' Takeda Pharmaceuticals International, Inc., Takeda Pharmaceuticals, LLC, Takeda Global Research & Development Center, Inc., Takeda Pharmaceuticals U.S.A., Inc., Takeda Pharmaceuticals America, Inc. and Abbott Laboratories, Inc.'s Motion to Dismiss Counts I, V, VI, VII, VIII, IX, X, XI, XII, XIII, XIV, and Punitive Damage Claims of Plaintiffs' [sic] Amended Complaint (Document No. 12, filed June 20, 2012) ("Defendants' Motion to Dismiss") and Plaintiff David S. Tatum's Memorandum of Law in Opposition to Defendants' Motion to Dismiss (Document No. 15, filed July 19, 2012), **IT IS ORDERED** that Defendants' Motion to Dismiss is **GRANTED IN PART AND DENIED IN PART** as follows:

1. Defendants' Motion to Dismiss is **GRANTED** with respect to Count I—equitable tolling of applicable statute of limitations; Count IX—strict product liability: defective design; Count XI—strict product liability: failure to warn; and Count XIII—unjust enrichment; and all such claims are **DISMISSED WITH PREJUDICE.**

2. Defendants' Motion to Dismiss is **DENIED** with respect to the remaining claims: Count V—negligent misrepresentation; Count VI—breach of express warranty; Count VII—breach of implied warranty for a particular purpose; Count VIII—breach of implied warranty of merchantability; Count X—strict product liability: manufacturing defect; Count XII—fraudulent concealment; and Count XIV—violations of Pennsylvania Unfair Trade Practices and Consumer Protection Law.

3. Defendants' Motion to Dismiss is **DENIED** with respect to plaintiff's request for punitive damages.

IT IS FURTHER ORDERED that a preliminary pretrial conference will be scheduled in due course.

THE FOLLOWING IS **the original unedited version**

IN THE UNITED STATES DISTRICT COURT FOR THE EASTERN DISTRICT OF PENNSYLVANIA

_________________________________ DAVID S. TATUM, :

Plaintiff, : v. :

TAKEDA PHARMACEUTICALS : NORTH AMERICA, INC., TAKEDA : PHARMACEUTICALS AMERICA, INC., TAKEDA PHARMACEUTICALS : INTERNATIONAL, INC., TAKEDA PHARMACEUTICALS COMPANY LIMITED, TAKEDA PHAR-MACEUTICALS, LLC, TAKEDA AMERICA HOLDINGS, INC., TAKEDA GLOBAL RESEARCH & : DEVELOPMENT CENTER, INC.,

TAKEDA SAN DIEGO, INC., TAP PHARMACEUTICALS PRODUCTS, INC., ABBOTT LABORATORIES, INC., DOES 1 THROUGH 100 INCLUSIVE,

Defendants. _________________________________

DuBois, J.

I. INTRODUCTION

CIVIL ACTION NO. 12-1114

MEMORANDUM

October 18, 2012

This is a product liability action in which plaintiff David S. Tatum alleges that the PREVACID designed, manufactured, and marketed by defendants weakened his bones, ultimately leading to hip fractures. The defendants filed a motion to dismiss many of the claims in Tatum's First Amended Complaint. For the reasons that follow, the Court grants in part and denies in part defendants' motion.

II. BACKGROUND 1

Tatum was prescribed PREVACID, a pharmaceutical drug designed, manufactured, and marketed by defendants. (Am. Compl. 3, 7.) After taking PREVACID, Tatum began feeling pain in his left hip, and he was later diagnosed with Stage III Avascular Necrosis. (Id. at 7.) Tatum's bones became weakened or brittle, causing multiple fractures. (Id. at 8.) As a result, he underwent total hip replacement surgery. (Id. at 7.)

Tatum claims that defendants were aware of the risks of PREVACID, but chose not to disclose them. His First Amended Complaint contains fourteen counts: Count I – equitable tolling of applicable statute of limitations; Count II – negligence; Count III – negligent failure to adequately warn; Count IV – negligence per se; Count V – negligent misrepresentation; Count VI – breach of express warranty; Count VII – breach of implied warranty for a particular purpose; Count VIII – breach of implied warranty of merchantability; Count IX – strict product liability: defective design; Count X – strict product liability: manufacturing defect; Count XI – strict product liability: failure to warn; Count XII – fraudulent concealment; Count XIII – unjust enrichment; and Count XIV – violations of Pennsylvania Unfair Trade Practices and Consumer Protection Law. Tatum additionally alleges that he is entitled to punitive damages.

Defendants have moved to dismiss Count I, Counts V to XIV, and the request for punitive damages.

1 As required on a motion to dismiss, the Court takes all plausible factual allegations contained in plaintiff's First Amended Complaint to be true.

III. STANDARD OF REVIEW

To survive a motion to dismiss under Rule 12(b)(6), a civil plaintiff must allege facts that "'raise a right to relief above the speculative level.'" Victaulic Co. v. Tieman, 499 F.3d 227, 234 (3d Cir. 2007) (quoting Bell Atl. Corp. v. Twombly, 550 U.S. 544, 555 (2007)). A complaint must contain "sufficient factual matter, accepted as true, to 'state a claim to relief that is plausible on its face.'" Ashcroft v. Iqbal, 556 U.S. 662, 678 (2009) (quoting Twombly, 550 U.S. at 570). "[T]he tenet that a court must accept as true all of the allegations contained in a complaint is inapplicable to legal conclusions. Threadbare recitals of the elements of a cause of action, supported by mere conclusory statements, do not suffice." Id.

IV. DISCUSSION

Defendants have moved to dismiss eleven of the fourteen counts in the First Amended Complaint, in addition to Tatum's request for punitive damages. The Court will address each in turn.

A. Count I: Equitable Tolling

Defendants initially move to dismiss Tatum's claim for equitable tolling alleged in Count I. Tatum alleges that "[t]he running of any statute of limitations has been tolled by reason of Defendants' fraudulent concealment." (Am. Compl. 11.) Fraudulent concealment is a doctrine which "serves to toll the running of the statute of limitations." Fine v. Checcio, 582 Pa. 253, 271 (2005). Unlike the tort of fraudulent concealment alleged in Count XII, this doctrine is not an independent cause of action. Thus, Count I is dismissed with prejudice.

It appears that by moving to dismiss Count I, defendants are also attempting to attack Tatum's tort claims, which are subject to a two-year statute of limitations. See 42 PA. CONS. STAT. ANN. § 5524; Mest v. Cabot Corp., 449 F.3d 502, 510 (2006). Generally, "a limitations defense must be raised in the answer, since Rule 12(b) does not permit it to be raised by motion." Robinson v. Johnson, 313 F.3d 128, 134 (3d Cir. 2002). However, the "Third Circuit Rule" allows defendants to raise a limitations defense in a Rule 12(b)(6) motion where the "time alleged in the statement of a claim shows that the cause of action has not been brought within the statute of limitations." Id. at 135.

Tatum filed his initial Complaint on March 1, 2012. (Compl. 35.) In his First Amended Complaint, he states that "[a]t no point prior to March 2010 had Plaintiff experienced any type of abnormal hip pain . . . ." (Am. Compl. 7.) As this allegation falls within the two-year period, the Court will not dismiss any claims on statute of limitations grounds on the present state of the record.

B. Counts IX, X, and XI: Strict Liability Claims

The Court next addresses Tatum's strict liability claims. Counts IX and XI which assert claims or strict liability based on design defect and strict liability based on failure to warn are not permitted under Pennsylvania law. Applying comment k to § 402A of the Restatement (Second) of Torts, the Pennsylvania Supreme Court ruled that "where the adequacy of warnings associated with prescription drugs is at issue, the failure of the manufacturer to exercise reasonable care to warn of dangers, i.e., the manufacturer's negligence, is the only recognized basis of liability." Hahn v. Richter, 543 Pa. 558, 563 (1996). As a result, Tatum cannot bring strict liability claims for design defect or failure to warn.

Count X which alleges a claim of strict liability based on manufacturing defect, however, is permissible. Many courts have interpreted Hahn broadly to preclude all strict liability claims. See Doughtery v. C.R. Bard, Inc., No. 11-6048, 2012 WL 2940727, at *4 (E.D. Pa. July 18, 2012) (collecting cases). However, this Court agrees with the decision in Doughtery, where the court concluded that strict liability claims for manufacturing defects are not prohibited. See id. at *4-6; Killen v. Stryker Spine, No. 11-1508, 2012 WL 4498865, at *3-4 (W.D. Pa. Sept. 28, 2012).

Tatum's claims in Count IX for strict liability based on design defect and Count XI for strict liability based on failure to warn are dismissed with prejudice. The strict liability claim based on manufacturing defect asserted in Count X is permitted under Pennsylvania Law. Thus, the motion to dismiss with respect to the claim for strict liability based on manufacturing defect asserted in Count X is denied.

C. Counts VI, VII, and VIII: Breach of Warranty Claims

Defendants further move to dismiss Tatum's breach of warranty claims. In his First Amended Complaint, Tatum alleges breach of implied warranty of merchantability

in Count VIII, breach of implied warranty for a particular purpose in Count VII, and breach of express warranty in Count VI.

(a) Counts VII and VIII: Breach of Implied Warranty of Fitness for a Particular Purpose and Breach of Implied Warranty of Merchantability

"[T]he theories of strict liability and breach of the implied warranty of merchantability are parallel theories of recovery, one in contract and the other in tort." Doughtery, 2012 WL 2940727 at *7 (internal quotations omitted). As discussed above, strict liability claims based on design defect or failure to warn are not permissible in Pennsylvania. "It would thus be inconsistent to exempt a manufacturer . . . from strict liability under comment k and apply a negligence standard to determine liability for a design defect or a failure to warn, but allow a plaintiff to recover for the same alleged defect under a theory of breach of the implied warranty of merchantability." Id. The same analysis applies to the implied warranty of fitness for a particular purpose. Both claims are not cognizable under Pennsylvania law to the extent they are based on a design defect or failure to warn, but are permissible if based on manufacturing defect or any other theory. Thus, the motion to dismiss with respect to the claims, as limited by this Memorandum, for breach of the implied warranty fitness for a particular purpose asserted in

Count VII and for breach of the implied warranty of merchantability asserted in Count VIII is denied.

(b) Count VI: Breach of Express Warranty

Tatum's remaining breach of warranty claim is for breach of express warranty. Federal courts are split concerning whether an express warranty claim against prescription drug manufacturers is permissible under Pennsylvania law. Id. (collecting cases). This Court concludes that such a claim is permitted. "While the reasoning of comment k may prevent certain warranties or promises from being implied by law," that is not a "basis for declining to enforce a contractual promise expressly and voluntarily made by a manufacturer of prescription drugs or devices." Id. Thus, the motion to dismiss with respect to the claim for breach of an express warranty asserted in Count VI is denied.

D. Count V: Negligent Misrepresentation

Defendants additionally move to dismiss Tatum's claim for negligent misrepresentation alleged in Count V because Tatum failed to allege his claim with the particularity required by Federal Rule of Civil Procedure 9(b). Although a plaintiff must plead negligent misrepresentation with a degree of specificity, Rule 9(b) does not govern negligent misrepresentation claims. Brandow Chrysler Jeep Co. v. DataScan Techs. 511 F.Supp.2d 529, 537 (E.D. Pa. 2007); but see Scott v. Bimbo Bakeries, USA, Inc., 2012 WL 645905, at *5 (E.D. Pa. Feb. 29, 2012) (noting "that there is disagreement among the district courts within the Third Circuit regarding the pleading standard that applies to claims of negligent misrepresentation."). Tatum alleges that defendants falsely represented "that PREVACID was safe and fit for its intended purpose, was of merchantable quality, did not produce any dangerous side effects, and had been adequately tested." (Am. Compl. 18.) This is a sufficiently specific allegation. Thus, the motion to dismiss with respect to the claim for negligent misrepresentation asserted in Count V is denied.

E. Counts XII and XIV: Fraudulent Concealment and Violations of Pennsylvania's Unfair Trade Practices and Consumer Protection Law

Defendants next move to dismiss Tatum's claims for fraudulent concealment alleged in Count XII and for violations of Pennsylvania's Unfair Trade Practices and Consumer Protection Law, 73 PA. CONS. STAT. ANN. §§ 201-1 et seq. (UTPCPL) alleged in Count XIV. Fraudulent concealment "has the same elements as intentional misrepresentation except in the case of intentional non-disclosure, the party intentionally conceals a material fact rather than making an affirmative misrepresentation." Bortz v. Noon, 556 Pa. 489, 499 (1999) (internal quotations omitted).2

Section 201-3 of the UTPCPL makes "[u]nfair methods of competition and unfair or deceptive acts or practices in the conduct of any trade or commerce . . . unlawful." Section 201-2(4)(xxi), the so- called "catch-all" definition, defines "[u]nfair methods of competition and unfair or deceptive acts or practices" as "[e]ngaging in any other fraudulent or deceptive conduct which creates a likelihood of confusion or of misunderstanding." "A plaintiff may succeed under the catch-all provision by satisfying the elements of common-law fraud." Vassalotti v. Wells Fargo Bank, N.A. 732 F.Supp.2d 503 (E.D. Pa 2010). The fraud can be based on the intentional concealment of information. Meeks-Owens v. Indymac Bank, F.S.B., 557 F.Supp.2d 566, 579 (M.D. Pa. 2008). Thus, Tatum's claims for fraudulent concealment and for violations of the UTPCPL overlap.

Defendants argue that both claims, which are based on intentional conduct, should be dismissed because they "do not rest on a theory of negligence." (Def. Mot. 12.) For this proposition, defendants cite the Pennsylvania Supreme Court's statement in Hahn that "where the adequacy of warnings associated with prescription drugs is at issue, the failure of the manufacturer to exercise reasonable care to warn of dangers, i.e., the manufacturer's negligence, is the only recognized basis of liability." 543 Pa. at 563.

This Court disagrees. The court in Hahn stated that a seller of prescription drugs must not only warn of risks of which he reasonably should have knowledge, but also warn of risks of which he did, in fact, have knowledge. Id. at 561. Accordingly, Hahn does not preclude claims where the plaintiff alleges that the seller had knowledge of the risks of prescription drugs and intentionally concealed them.

For this reason, the motion to dismiss with respect to the claims for fraudulent concealment asserted in Count XII and for violations of Pennsylvania's Unfair Trade Practices and Consumer Protection Law asserted in Count XIV is denied. Since Tatum has stated a claim under the "fraud prong" of the catch- all provision of the UTPCPL, the Court does not address the "deceptive conduct" prong of the catch-all provision or the other provisions of the UPTCPL referenced in the First Amended Complaint.

2 The elements of intentional misrepresentation or fraud are: "(1) A representation; (2) which is material to the transaction at hand; (3) made falsely, with knowledge of its falsity or recklessness as to whether it is true or false; (4) with the intent of misleading another into relying on it; (5) justifiable reliance on the misrepresentation; and, (6) the resulting injury was proximately caused by the reliance." Id.

F. Count XIII: Unjust Enrichment

Defendants also move to dismiss Tatum's claim for unjust enrichment alleged in Count XIII. "Under Pennsylvania law, the plaintiff must demonstrate that he conferred a benefit on the defendant, that the defendant knew of the benefit and accepted or retained it, and that it would be inequitable to allow the defendant to keep the benefit without paying for it." Zafarana, 724 F.Supp. 2d at 560. However, "[u]njust enrichment is not a substitute for failed tort claims in Pennsylvania . . . ." Id. (internal citations omitted).

This is not a case in which a claim for unjust enrichment is appropriate. Specifically, there is no allegation that defendants refused to provide a service or goods after Tatum provided defendants with a benefit. See id. at 561. Thus, Tatum's claim in Count XIII for unjust enrichment is dismissed with prejudice.

G. Punitive Damages

Finally, defendants move to dismiss Tatum's request for punitive damages. Defendants argue that under Pennsylvania law, punitive damages are not an independent cause of action. Kirkbride v. Lisbon Contractors, Inc., 521 Pa. 97, 101 (1989). That is correct. However, Tatum did not assert an independent claim for punitive damages in the First Amended Complaint. Rather, he requested punitive damages as a remedy. Punitive damages are properly alleged in the First Amended Complaint.

V . CONCLUSION

For the reasons set forth above, the Court grants in part and denies in part defendants' motion to dismiss. Count I – equitable tolling of applicable statute of limitations; Count IX – strict product liability: defective design; Count XI – strict product liability: failure to warn; and Count XIII – unjust enrichment; are dismissed with prejudice.

The claims remaining for adjudication are: Count V – negligent misrepresentation; Count VI – breach of express warranty; Count VII – breach of implied warranty for a particular purpose; Count VIII – breach of implied warranty of merchantability; Count X – strict product liability: manufacturing defect; Count XII – fraudulent concealment; and Count XIV – violations of Pennsylvania Unfair Trade Practices and Consumer Protection Law.

The Court concludes that many of Tatum's remaining claims are redundant or otherwise unnecessary, making this case unduly complicated. At the preliminary pretrial conference, the Court will address narrowing the scope of the issues presented.

An appropriate order follows.

· · ·

UNITED STATES DISTRICT COURT,

E.D. Pennsylvania.

David S. TATUM, Plaintiff,

v.

TAKEDA PHARMACEUTICALS NORTH AMERICA, INC., Takeda Pharmaceuticals America, Inc., Takeda Pharmaceuticals International, Inc., Takeda Pharmaceuticals Company Limited, Takeda Pharmaceuticals, LLC, Takeda America Holdings, Inc., Takeda Global Research & Development Center, Inc., Takeda San Diego, Inc., Tap Pharmaceuticals Products, Inc., Abbott Laboratories, Inc., Does 1 through 100 Inclusive, Defendants.

Civil Action No. 12–1114.

Oct. 19, 2012.

Attorneys and Law Firms

Claudine Q. Homolash, Sheller P.C., Philadelphia, PA, Kenneth G. Gilman, Gilman Law LLP, Bonita Springs, FL, for Plaintiff.

Tiffany M. Alexander, Campbell Campbell Edwards & Conroy, Wayne, PA, for Defendants.

ORDER

JAN E. DuBOIS, District Judge.

***1 AND NOW,** this 18th day of October, 2012, upon consideration of Defendants' Takeda Pharmaceuticals International, Inc., Takeda Pharmaceuticals, LLC, Takeda Global Research & Development Center, Inc., Takeda Pharmaceuticals U.S.A., Inc., Takeda Pharmaceuticals America, Inc. and Abbott Laboratories, Inc.'s Motion to Dismiss Counts I, V, VI, VII, VIII, IX, X, XI, XII, XIII, XIV, and Punitive Damage Claims of Plaintiffs' [sic] Amended Complaint (Document No. 12, filed June 20, 2012) ("Defendants' Motion to Dismiss") and Plaintiff David S. Tatum's Memorandum of Law in Opposition to Defendants' Motion to Dismiss (Document No. 15, filed July 19, 2012), **IT IS ORDERED** that Defendants' Motion to Dismiss is **GRANTED IN PART AND DENIED IN PART** as follows:

1. Defendants' Motion to Dismiss is **GRANTED** with respect to Count I—equitable tolling of applicable statute of limitations; Count IX—strict product liability: defective design; Count XI—strict product liability: failure to warn; and Count XIII—unjust enrichment; and all such claims are **DISMISSED WITH PREJUDICE.**

2. Defendants' Motion to Dismiss is **DENIED** with respect to the remaining claims: Count V—negligent misrepresentation; Count VI—breach of express warranty; Count VII—breach of implied warranty for a particular purpose; Count VIII—breach of implied warranty of merchantability; Count X—strict product liability: manufacturing defect; Count XII—fraudulent concealment; and Count XIV—violations of Pennsylvania Unfair Trade Practices and Consumer Protection Law.

3. Defendants' Motion to Dismiss is **DENIED** with respect to plaintiff's request for punitive damages.

IT IS FURTHER ORDERED that a preliminary pretrial conference will be scheduled in due course.

11

BECOMING A WHISTLEBLOWER

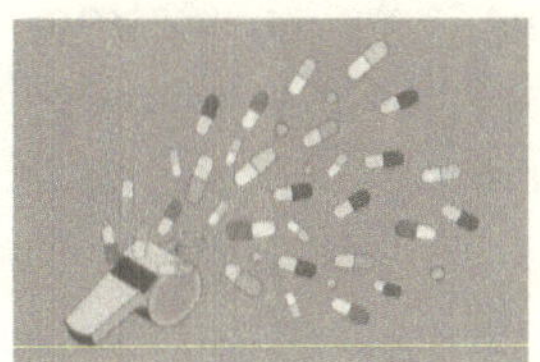

The New England Journal of Medicine is one of the most respected medical journals around the globe. A 2010 article titled, "Whistle-Blowers' Experiences in Fraud Litigation against Pharmaceutical Companies"[1] by Aaron S. Kesselheim, MD et al. was a wealth of specific information.

A significant question is, what motivates an employee to become a whistleblower? The NEJM's study identified four elements that explain why employees blow the whistle: Self-preservation, Justice, Integrity, and Altruism or Public Safety.

Of the twenty-six pharmaceutical whistleblowers they interviewed for the article, only six began the process intending to do so. The other twenty were encouraged to share their information by attorneys they reached out to for different reasons.

The most common trait, in 11 of the 26, was integrity and wanting to do the right thing. An attribute existing in 7 of the 26 relators was trying to prevent public health risks, but it didn't say how many of the 26 were in a situation where health concerns were an issue.

The personal toll experienced by the whistleblowers was an issue with most of them. Not only was it a career-limiting move, but also had "devastating" financial consequences for at least 8 of the 26. Six of the 26 reported divorces and other severe marital issues while thirteen reported stress-related medical issues including, "shingles, psoriasis, autoimmune disorders, panic attacks, asthma, insomnia, temporomandibular joint disorder, migraine headaches, and generalized anxiety."

An important thing to walk away from the study with is that 22 of the 26 relators felt that, "what they did was important for ethical and other psychological or spiritual reasons."

I would have to say that this article is spot on in many ways. I was not planning on being a whistleblower until speaking with lawyers about another concern. I was trying to prevent a public health risk involving double dosing a product that has a warning in its package insert to use the lowest dose possible for the shortest duration. It was a definite career limiting move, not limited to the company, but expanding to the industry as a whole due to the availability of information via the internet. Although I didn't have the stress-related issues described I did experience severe stress and depression throughout the roller coaster of ups and downs during the process. My marriage of almost fourteen years ended during the years of the case.

While talking to lawyers, they suggested that pharmaceutical companies often do off-label things. That is what made me think of how Takeda only promotes Dexilant at 60mg when patients should just be on 30mg, at least start on 30mg.

I mentioned this earlier in the book, but it is an excellent point to revisit the story. In the book "GRIT – The Power of Passion and Perseverance"[2] by Angela Duckworth she refers to a parable about three workers building a church that stuck with me. When asked what they do, the first worker replied that he has a job as a bricklayer. The second worker replied that he is a bricklayer constructing a building. The third worker said that he is a bricklayer building a house of God. The bricklayers viewed what they do as a job, a career, and a calling.

To take this one step further, which is not what the author's intention was, but imagine how the third worker who saw laying bricks for the church as a calling would feel if he discovered that the foreman used lower standard materials to increase profits. Now imagine what if by using the lower quality materials a safety issue arose seriously injuring worshippers during a wedding or funeral service. How does that change how you feel?

There are so many factors that made the lawsuits possible and I realize that without having an attorney in the family, along with good friends that had their own law practice, none of this would have come to light. Hopefully, companies will not look at employees with attorneys in the family as a liability, but only seek to obey the law.

My good friends from Bell & Bell LLP, along with my wife at the time, all three Georgetown University Law School graduates, looked into our options and we decided to have Bell & Bell LLP handle the case.

Once we knew what needed to be done they prepared the legal documents and began the process. Because the issue was so obvious, when you knew what you were looking for, we thought that we wouldn't be the first to file the *qui tam*, especially regarding the promotion to rheumatologists.

The issue with rheumatologists is that Prevacid had two indications for NSAID use; one for Healing NSAID associated gastric ulcers and one for maintaining healed NSAID associated gastric related ulcers. Dexilant does not have any NSAID indications, and thus representatives should not have been permitted to promote it to rheumatologists since they would not be prescribing it for GERD. Since Takeda was trying to recoup the $3 billion Prevacid market we were calling on almost anyone that was writing Prevacid and trying to get them to switch their patients over to Dexilant. And yes, representatives were explicitly being paid for Dexilant prescriptions being written by rheumatologists and rheumatologists were ranked on a 1-10 scale for their importance to prescribing Dexilant.

We filed the False Claims Act Complaint in July 2009 in the Eastern District of Pennsylvania. We became very excited when the Department of Justice contacted us about the case after only a short period of time. Since I lived in Virginia, they asked for the case to be transferred down to the Eastern District of Virginia, and we agreed. The initial meeting was at FBI Headquarters on October 30, 2009, in Washington, DC where government lawyers and agents interviewed me at a huge rectangular table. At the meeting were special agents from the FBI, the FDA, and Health and Human Services along with attorneys from the United States Attorney Office of the Eastern District of Virginia Criminal, United States Attorney Office of the Eastern District of Virginia Civil, and a trial attorney from the United States Department of Justice.

I was asked a lot of questions during the meeting, and the government came well prepared. The FDA agent was explaining to the table how Dexilant is the R-enantiomer of Prevacid (lansoprazole). Think of your left and right hands, they mirror each other but are not the same. Think of Dexilant as the right hand of Prevacid along with a dual delayed release (DDR) technology to make one pill work as two.

We went through a lot of our initial complaint that we filed with the Department of Justice, and they were very enthusiastic about it. They asked me if I would be willing to wear a wire if the opportunity presented itself? I said I would.

The agents did most of the questioning, but the lawyers were very interested because they would be the ones to take the case to court. Government attorneys only take a small percentage of *qui tam* cases due to their caseload abilities.

The meeting went very well, and it led to two FBI special agents and an FDA special agent accompanying me to a sales meeting in Phoenix, Arizona. At this point, the case was still under seal, so Takeda was not aware of my actions. (I describe wearing a wire for the government at that meeting in a later chapter)

Having read his book for research, Stephen Martin Kohn is known as one of the top whistleblower attorneys in the United States. He is the founding partner of Kohn, Kohn, and Colapinto, LLP in Washington DC. In 1988 he helped establish the National Whistleblower Center where he currently serves as the Executive Director.

"The New Whistleblower's Handbook: A Step-By-Step Guide To Doing What's Right And Protecting Yourself"[3] by Stephen Martin Kohn

I gained a lot of useful information from Kohn's book, and if you are reading my book debating whether or not to be a whistleblower yourself, I would highly recommend it. His book will inform you for what needs to be done and what you need to prepare yourself for. Kohn explains, "It was determined that whistleblowers are the single most effective source of information in both detecting and rooting out corporate criminal activity." He shows that between 1986 and 2016 the government successfully prosecuted fraud cases and recovered over $15 billion. During the same time period, with the help of whistleblowers, the government recovered over $37 billion. Whistleblowers now uncover 70 percent of the civil frauds retrieved by the United States.

My primary motivation for what I did and why I am writing this book is because I tried to do the right thing. Since I was blocked from proving my case in the court of law, I will plead my case in the court of public opinion.

Kohn states that almost all employees tagged as whistleblowers were just doing their jobs. In the process of doing their jobs, they became aware of an issue, and they felt the need to bring in authorities to make it right. It is not a decision made lightly but one that is important enough to go through the process. The biggest issue is the David & Goliath dilemma. The employee with the knowledge of the wrongdoing wants to do the right thing, but they fear they will be helpless against the resourceful giant. We have all seen the movies where the big dominant company uses its leverage and high priced attorneys to push the little guy around, and they get away with it.

Takeda Pharmaceuticals is my Goliath, and they brought the high-priced New York City law firm of Patterson Belknap (pbwt.com). Their principal attorney was William F. Cavanaugh, Jr, a senior litigation partner who served as Co-Chair of the firm from 2007 - 2017, during the years of my case. They had the principal attorney plus several associates from a Big NYC firm against a small three-attorney firm from Philadelphia. My lawyers were great, but we were fighting an uphill battle in the 4th circuit. For our appeal, we reached out to an expert in this area and hired the law firm MoloLamken LLP from Washington, DC. Jeff Lamken and Michael Pattillo Jr. took the case through the uphill battle of the 4th circuit and up to the Supreme Court of the United States. Their argument was so compelling that organizations which cover the Supreme Court thought my case would be accepted to resolve the circuit split.

In a perfect system the right guy would always win, but unfortunately, the law is a very complicated process. I like to look at it as playing chess, and your opponent isn't familiar with the move "En Passant." En Passant is a move a player can use when their opponent advances a pawn the allowed two spaces, as that pawn's initial move. However, if moving only a single space would have left them open to an opposing pawn, then that opposing pawn can use the rule to take the piece. This rule is straight-forward, but if you were not aware of the rule it would seem like cheating. Since the law is not as clear and is up for interpretation, it can be just as frustrating.

Cases are not won because they are right, they are won by being able to check the required boxes and provide enough evidence to prove the case, even if your hands are tied in the process. I have talked about it before, but if I was able to show the data I had, which only became available after the case began, about my physicians writing Dexilant at the 60mg strength, their argument that I couldn't show any prescriptions were written goes away. So, to win a case, on top of being right, knowing the rules, having people putting themselves at risk to do the right thing, and having the financial ability to fight the case, I am adding timing to the equation. As I will get into later in the book, a significant factor in winning a court case is which judge you get and where the lawsuit is filed. Regarding the False Claims Act, I will have a considerable ask, but you need more information first.

On that same idea, the opposition is trying to win by pointing out that boxes aren't checked and arguing that the boxes that are claimed to be checked, should not be allowed. I lost my case before being able to get to a trial to prove my facts. I lost at the "motion to dismiss" phase of the process.

Most employees will report the controversial issue to their manager, or along the chain of authority depending on the situation. It is important to remember that the employee is exposing himself by reporting the issue and that the person to whom you are communicating might have the safety of the company as their main priority, thereby stopping the employee could be beneficial to that end.

From my experience, I didn't have any confidence that reporting the off-label double dosing of Dexilant would be taken seriously.

Self-preservation is a natural human reflex, and an employee must keep it in mind before they come forward with a potential whistleblower complaint. In a perfect world, everyone would be working together to do the right thing and to keep society safe. Since that is not the reality we live in, it is imperative that the brave people willing to take the risk to do the right thing protect themselves.

The company officials you tell about the issue might try and keep you quiet by changing your job, ignoring your claim, terminating you from the organization, or even blaming you for the problem. In my case, I was moved off of selling Dexilant about a year after Takeda became aware of my involvement. I was moved to another medication to promote, ending my ability to access Dexilant sales data.

It is imperative to cover your ass before you relate what you know to the company. Lawyers working for the company, as well as those hired by the company, are single-focused to protect their client. They might try and get around the ethical issue by stopping the client from informing them of specific knowledge, to claim they didn't know, but we have all seen this scenario before.

Kohn points out that there is a difference between company compliance programs which report to their lawyers, compared to the company compliance programs that report directly to the CEO or Board of Directors. Experts in the area of compliance argue that a General Counsel (attorney) in charge of compliance programs is a bad idea because of the need for transparency, independence, and to build trust. Company lawyers can use the attorney-client privilege to hide information critical to an investigation. Kohn's research shows that in a March 2013 survey of ten thousand compliance professionals, 88.5% were opposed to the company's general counsel serving as the compliance officer. They recognized the conflict of interest between the two positions, and the issues that could arise between encouraging employees to report wrongdoing and defending against them.

The 1986 amendments to the False Claims Act added protections for the whistleblower from retaliation. The 1986 addition includes termination and job discrimination against any employee who files or assists with an FCA investigation. It allows for employees to be reinstated, receive double back pay, have their attorney fees paid, and the potential of special damages. Kohn shows that the whistleblower's career and reputation will be damaged and "is often completely destroyed." It is tough to fight companies in whistleblower cases, and it is just as hard, if not harder, to fight for being terminated as retaliation.

According to Kohn, it is almost impossible to defeat a claim of poor performance as a reason for termination. The company has incredible resources including documents and employees that could be in fear of their own positions. Companies will not admit to firing employees in retaliation but will take time and build a case against them based on poor performance. Courts have expressed how difficult it can be for employees to prove that "their protected activities caused their termination."

As with any litigation, having the ability to prove your case is critical. In pharmaceutical cases, it is becoming more challenging to acquire the evidence because of newer HIPAA standards. HIPAA stands for Health Insurance Portability and Accountability Act, and it increases the protection of personal patient information. Courts have established how data can be obtained for use to make sure employees didn't break any laws. The information I have was given to me as a representative working for Takeda.

The government has many resources and legal means to keep companies honest, but that doesn't mean they will be enacted. When we say "the government" we are really saying the individuals that are working for the government. Just like a federal law is different depending on where you are in the country, so are individual employees. The FCA whistleblower provision is still one of the most effective ways of protecting our government from fraud. An added benefit of the FCA is that companies are encouraged to remain honest from the threat of an employee turning them in for the reward. As the defense attorney John T. Boese states, "the FCA encourages adoption of best practices."

12

HISTORY OF THE FALSE CLAIMS ACT

The first whistleblowers in the United States, according to Stephen M. Kohn[1], were ten men comprised of six Navy and Marine Corps officers, three enlisted Naval sailors, and a military Chaplain speaking up against a Naval officer during the American Revolutionary War. Commodore Esek Hopkins was the highest ranked Naval officer, who also happened to be an attorney, and the whistleblowers informed Congress about his treatment of prisoners, his failure to attack a British ship, and his statement that he would not obey Congress. Their petition to Congress follows[2]:

On Board the Ship ' Warren ' Feb 19, 1777, Much Respected Gentlemen: "We who present this petition engaged on board the ship ' Warren ' with an earnest desire and fixed expectation of doing our country some service . . . . We are ready to hazard everything that is dear & if necessary, sacrifice our lives for the welfare of our country, we are desirous of being active in the defense of our constitutional liberties and privileges against the unjust cruel claims of tyranny & oppression; but as things are now circumstanced on board this frigate, there seems to be no prospect of our being serviceable in our present situation . . . . We are personally well acquainted with the real character & conduct of our commander, Commodore Hopkins & we take this method not having a more convenient opportunity of sincerely & humbly petitioning, the honorable Marine Committee that they would inquire into his character & conduct, for we suppose that his character is such & that he has been guilty of such crimes as render him quite unfit for the public department he now occupies, which crimes, we the subscribers can sufficiently attest. Each sailor also signed personal affidavits to Congress setting forth specific instances of misconduct committed by the commander in chief that they had witnessed. These included allegations that commodore Hopkins "treated prisoners in the most inhuman & barbarous manner, "failed to attack a British frigate that had run aground (thereby permitting the enemy to escape), and stated that he would "not obey the Congress."

CONGRESS LISTENED, investigated, and acted by suspending Commodore Hopkins from the Navy. It is important to remember that this was during the Revolutionary War and the Bill of Rights didn't exist. Kohn points out there was no First Amendment protection for freedom of speech or any legal protections for whistleblowers. Although Hopkins was removed from his command, he didn't go away quietly. Esek Hopkins was an attorney and wanted revenge. Before he was dismissed, Hopkins became aware of the investigation and about his subordinates who signed the petition. He used his authority to pressure his fellow officers to charge the signers with a crime. Hopkins ordered Lieutenant Marvin arrested and tried by a court-martial consisting of Hopkins' supporters including Hopkin's own son. If Lt. Marvin was found guilty his only appeal would be to Hopkins himself. Lt. Marvin was found guilty and expelled from the Navy.

Esek Hopkins was from Rhode Island, and since only two of the signers were in the jurisdiction of Rhode Island at the time, Lt. Richard Marvin and Midshipman Samuel Shaw were the only ones served with the complaint. Kohn provides that, "Shaw and Marvin were both arrested, held in jail, and forced to post an " enormous bail. "" The only place they could go for help was the Continental Congress. They petitioned Congress for help, and their petition was read to Congress on July 23, 1778. A special committee was appointed, and after a seven-day review, the committee reported back to the Congress on July 30, 1778, coming to the defense of Marvin and Shaw. Kohn states, "History was made. On July 30, 1778, the Continental Congress came to the defense of Marvin and Shaw. The Congress, without any recorded dissent, passed a resolution that encouraged all citizens to blow the whistle on official misconduct."

The Congressional Record-Senate shows on July 7, 2016[3]:

SENATE RESOLUTION 522—DESIGNATING JULY 30, 2016, AS "NATIONAL WHISTLEBLOWER APPRECIATION DAY"

Mr. GRASSLEY (for himself, Mr. WYDEN, Mr. KIRK, Mrs. MCCASKILL, Mr. JOHNSON, Mr. CARPER, Mrs. FISCHER, Ms. BALDWIN, Mr. TILLIS, Mr. MARKEY, Mrs. BOXER, Mrs. ERNST, Mr. PETERS, and Mr. BOOZMAN) submitted the following resolution; which was considered and agreed to:

S. RES. 522

Whereas, in 1777, before the passage of the Bill of Rights, 10 sailors and marines blew the whistle on fraud and misconduct harmful to the United States;

Whereas the Founding Fathers unanimously supported the whistleblowers in words and deeds, including by releasing government records and providing monetary assistance for reasonable legal expenses necessary to prevent retaliation against the whistleblowers;

Whereas, on July 30, 1778, in demonstration of their full support for whistleblowers, the members of the Continental Congress unanimously enacted the first whistleblower legislation in the United States that read: "Resolved, That it is the duty of all persons in the service of the United States, as well as all other the inhabitants thereof, to give the earliest information to Congress or other proper authority of any misconduct, frauds or misdemeanors committed by any officers or persons in the service of these states, which may come to their knowledge" (legislation of July 30, 1778, reprinted in Journals of the Continental Congress, 1774–1789, ed. Worthington C. Ford et al. (Washington, D.C., 1904–37), 11:732);

Whereas whistleblowers risk their careers, jobs, and reputations by reporting waste, fraud, and abuse to the proper authorities;

Whereas, when providing proper authorities with lawful disclosures, whistleblowers save taxpayers in the United States billions of dollars each year and serve the public interest by ensuring that the United States remains an ethical and safe place; and

Whereas it is the public policy of the United States to encourage, in accordance with Federal law (including the Constitution, rules, and regulations) and consistent with the protection of classified information (including sources and methods of detection of classified information), honest and good faith reporting of misconduct, fraud, misdemeanors, and other crimes to the appropriate authority at the earliest time possible: Now, therefore, be it Resolved, That the Senate—

(1) designates July 30, 2016, as "National Whistleblower Appreciation Day"; and

(2) ensures that the Federal Government implements the intent of the Founding Fathers, as reflected in the legislation enacted on July 30, 1778, by encouraging each executive agency to recognize National Whistleblower Appreciation Day by—

(A) informing employees, contractors working on behalf of United States taxpayers, and members of the public about the legal rights of citizens of the United States to "blow the whistle" by honest and good faith reporting of misconduct, fraud, misdemeanors, or other crimes to the appropriate authorities; and

(B) acknowledging the contributions of whistleblowers to combating waste, fraud, abuse, and violations of laws and regulations in the United States.

SUPREME COURT JUSTICE William O. Douglass stated in 1971, "The dominant purpose of the First Amendment was to prohibit the widespread practice of government suppression of embarrassing information." Kohn[4] provided this in his book and emphasized that "Whistleblowing embodies the heart and soul of the First Amendment. It establishes the right of the people to expose wrongdoing and empowers them with the right to demand that powerful leaders remain accountable."

Whistleblowing evolved and became more specific to encourage people with information to come forward and do the right thing. During the United States Civil War, President Lincoln signed the False Claims Act into law on March 2, 1863. This law was needed because government contractors were stealing from the U.S. Treasury by billing for inferior or non-existent goods.

The False Claims Act remains "the weapon of first choice in combating fraud in virtually every program involving federal funds," John T. Boese, Civil False Claims and Qui Tam Actions 1-5 (4th ed. 2011).[5]

The FCA has been amended five times since 1863. In 1986 Congress updated the False Claims Act to include a *qui tam* provision. *Qui tam* is short for "*qui tam pro domino rege quam pro se ipso in hac parte sequitur*," which translates to, "who pursues this action on our Lord the King's behalf as well as his own." With the update in 1986, it has proven to be the most effective antifraud law in the United States. Stephen M. Kohn shows, "The law is designed to encourage, protect, and reward employees who risk their careers to "do the right thing.""[6]

Under the FCA, any person who knowingly presents, or causes to be presented, a false or fraudulent claim for payment by the government, is liable for treble (triple) damages and penalties ranging from $5,000 to $10,000 for each claim.

The *qui tam* provision allows whistleblowers to file lawsuits to collect money on behalf of the government. For their efforts, the whistleblower would get a reward of 15 to 30 percent of the amount recovered plus they can be reimbursed for their legal fees during the process.

In 1943, Senator William Langer of North Dakota engaged in a filibuster to save the law. "I submit that the present statute now on the books is a most desirable one. What harm can there be if 10,000 lawyers in America are assisting the Attorney General of the United States in digging up war frauds? In any case, the Attorney General can protect himself by filing a (civil) lawsuit at the time when he files the indictment."[7] 89 Cong. Rec. 7607 (Sept. 17, 1943).

Luckily there are more organizations for than against doing the right thing. Kohn shows that "Even the most notorious anti-whistleblower business - lobbying group, the U.S. Chamber of Commerce Institute for Legal Reform, in a 2015 report, lauded the False Claims Act as "the government's most important tool to uncover and punish fraud against the United States."[8]

Attorney General Eric Holder stated, "The False Claims Act has provided ordinary Americans with essential tools to combat fraud, to help recover damages, and to bring accountability to those who would take advantage of the United States government and of American taxpayers."

"The False Claims Act works. It works because it is an effective tool to fight fraud across the full spectrum of federal programs and initiatives. The FCA works because it provides powerful incentives for companies to do business the right way."[9] Stuart Delery, Assistant U.S. Attorney General.

The False Claims Act does work. Since the update in 1986 more than $54 billion was collected by the United States plus over $6 billion was earned by whistleblowers. The actual benefit, which cannot be measured, is how companies have changed their practices due to the threat of being turned in. Companies created Ethics and Compliance departments, they have more oversight to make sure things are done correctly and have more transparency than in the past. These proactive measures not only save companies millions of dollars in legal liability but also lowers the risk to their reputation.

In 2009, the United States Congress added an amendment to the False Claims Act. On May 20, 2009, the Fraud Enforcement and Recovery Act (FERA) of 2009 was signed into law by President Obama. The FERA was in response to a U.S. Supreme Court decision in *Allison Engine Co. v. United States ex rel. Sanders.*[10]

Jeremy Gersh showed that Congress did not agree with the Supreme Court's decision in Allison Engine, and passed the amendment to clarify the law which the court will interpret in the future. "FERA completely rewrote § 3729 to return the statute to Congress's original intent. First, Congress rewrote § 3729(a)(2) by removing the phrase "paid or approved by the Government," and focused on "a false or fraudulent claim." Further, Congress added a materiality requirement to the FCA, defining materiality as "having a natural tendency to influence, or be capable of influencing, the payment or receipt of money or property." Now, a false statement only needs to be "material to a false or fraudulent claim," and there is no element of intent."[11]

MALCOLM GLADWELL IS a five-time New York Times bestselling author and host of his podcast, "Revisionist History." In his episode, "Burden of Proof" season 3 episode 2, Gladwell uses

Frederick Hoffman from 1918 as an example. Hoffman was a statistician with Prudential Life Insurance Company and noticed that coal miners were dying at an earlier age than the rest of the population. Trying to dispute his claim, some stated that coal miners have a lower rate of tuberculosis compared to others claiming the coal dust has a protective property. Hoffman didn't buy it and did his own research. He noted that coal miners did not have lower rates of tuberculosis while having five times the rates of asthma and death compared to the general population. Hoffman also stated that 1/3 of farmers were working past the age of 45 while only 1/5 of the coal miners were.[12]

Hoffman was so concerned about the issue that he wrote, "Mortality From Respiratory Diseases In Dusty Trades"[13] and it was published by the U.S. Department Of Labor Statistics in 1918. He was able to show the facts about the coal miners, but no one acted on it. The people who could have done something claimed there was only "suggestive evidence but no definitive evidence." It wasn't until the 1970's, over 50 years later, that the effects of coal dust were accepted.

This "suggestive evidence but no definitive evidence" is related to my whistleblower case which began in 2009 and ended in 2014 with the U.S. Supreme Court deciding not to take the appeal. The reason the Supreme Court was interested in my case was due to a significant circuit court split on a specific issue, Rule 9(b).

An interesting issue in the amendments from 1986 is that if an employee alleges an illegal scheme or action, the company must respond by conducting an investigation into the claim. During and after my complaint was made, Takeda never changed the way Dexilant was promoted. Remember, Dexilant 60mg is only indicated for "Healing of Erosive Esophagitis" "for up to 8 weeks". Takeda didn't change the policy of only sampling and promoting the 60 mg dose for years, and that was only on a limited basis where representatives were given some 30mg samples. A past-

President of the American Medical Association didn't know a 30mg dose was an option until after I contacted him about being an expert witness in my case. If, according to the 1986 update to the FCA, the company was supposed to investigate my claim, why didn't anything change?

In filing a *qui tam*, the whistleblower, known as the "relator," notifies the Department of Justice about the situation. The first step would be for the relator to obtain legal counsel and the attorney will file the necessary paperwork to begin the process. This process is filed "under seal" which means that the company is not aware of the action being filed. By keeping the process "under seal" it allows the government to investigate the accusation without tipping off the company and giving them the chance to cover their tracks. During this time the relator is not permitted to discuss the case except with their attorneys to make sure nothing is accidentally mentioned thus alerting the company. Imagine something that is such a huge part of your life, and you aren't allowed to discuss it outside of your legal counsel. During this period in my life, I gained a great appreciation of what members of our clandestine services must go through protecting us.

The time "under seal" is limited to allow the government time to decide if they want to enter the case. The government lawyers can choose to prosecute, or if they do not intervene, will enable the relator the option to litigate the case themselves or just drop the action entirely. Having the government enter a case is a huge deal. If the Department of Justice enters a whistle-blower case, the probability of winning or having the case settle is astronomical.

To show how important it is for the government to intervene, the following is from the U.S. Department of Justice Fraud Statistics regarding False Claims Act recoveries in Health-Care actions for the years 2012 to 2016. The government claims that failure to intervene is not necessarily related to the case but with the ability to manage the increasing caseload with 414 new qui tams filed in 2012 and 501 recorded in 2016:

2012 *Qui Tam* U.S. intervened $2.5 Billion
2012 *Qui Tam* U.S. declined to intervene$37.6 Million
2013 *Qui Tam* U.S. intervened$2.5 Billion
2013 *Qui Tam* U.S. declined to intervene$119 Million
2014 *Qui Tam* U.S. intervened$2.3 Billion
2014 *Qui Tam* U.S. declined to intervene$66 Million
2015 *Qui Tam* U.S. intervened$1.5 Billion
2015 *Qui Tam* U.S. declined to intervene$472.6 Million
2016 *Qui Tam* U.S. intervened$2.4 Billion
2016 *Qui Tam* U.S. declined to intervene$72 Million

IN AN ARTICLE by David Pivnick of FCA Insider[14], he explains that the number of whistleblower cases filed has nearly doubled in the years from 2008 to 2014. He shows that government intervention is less than 25 percent of the cases filed and over 90 percent of the recoveries come from those cases.

An article by Amandeep S. Sidhu on December 9, 2014, from the "Health Law Litigation,"[15] shows that government intervention is significant and that 94 percent of cases where the government did not intervene were dismissed.

The following paragraph is a critical part of this book and my case. Since it pertains to several areas and ideas of the book, I feel the need to state it throughout. As we showed in our Supreme Court Cert Petition:

WHETHER RULE 9(b) requires that a complaint under the False Claims Act "allege with particularity that specific false claims actually were presented to the government for payment," as required by the Fourth, Sixth, Eighth, and Eleventh Circuits, or whether it is instead sufficient to allege the "particular details of" the "scheme to submit false claims" together with sufficient indicia that false claims were submitted, as held by the First, Fifth, Seventh, and Ninth Circuits.

UNFORTUNATELY, it is vital where you file a federal case. Federal law should be the same throughout the country, but as I show, there is a sharp circuit court split on how to interpret specific portions of federal law. We submitted our Complaint on September 14, 2009, in the Federal Eastern District of Pennsylvania, which is where my attorneys at Bell & Bell LLP are located. The Federal Eastern District of Pennsylvania is in Philadelphia, PA, which is in the Federal 3rd Circuit. The Federal 3rd Circuit has had pharmaceutical *qui tam* experience and were not part of Rule 9(b) divide, but that wasn't a concern at the time of the filing. Since I lived in Virginia, the Eastern District of Virginia office asked to have the case transferred, and we agreed. By moving the case, we came under the jurisdiction of the Federal 4th Circuit and their version of federal law interpretation.

13

RHEUMATOLOGISTS

When this process began, we thought the rheumatologist part of the complaint was going to be the easiest of any of the issues we presented since it was so obvious. Dexilant 60mg was only indicated for erosive esophagitis for 8 weeks, and there is no reason why a rheumatologist would ever diagnose erosions of the throat.

According to the American College of Rheumatology[1], a rheumatologist treats diseases that can affect the joints, muscles, and bones which can cause pain, swelling, stiffness, and deformity in the patient.

Prevacid was the first PPI approved for both Healing NSAID associated gastric ulcers and Risk Reduction of NSAID associated gastric ulcers in December 2000. NSAIDs are Non-Steroidal Anti-Inflammatory Drugs such as aspirin, ibuprofen (Advil), and naproxen (Aleve) to name a few. NSAIDs are used for minor aches and pains such as headaches, muscle pain, joint pain, backaches, and arthritis. They are mostly over the counter (OTC) medications and one of the most widely used classes of drugs in the United States with billions of uses annually. The downside is that NSAIDs interfere with the protective lining of the stomach and can lead to NSAID associated gastric ulcers.

An explanation of how NSAIDs work from the medical journal, *Best Practice & Research Clinical Gastroenterology*[2], Dr. C.J. Hawkey explains that, "By inhibiting prostaglandin synthesis, non-steroidal anti-inflammatory drugs (NSAIDs) cause mucosal damage, ulceration and ulcer complication throughout the gastrointestinal tract. The recognition that there are two cyclooxygenase enzymes, one predominating at sites of inflammation (COX-2) and one constitutively expressed in the gastrointestinal tract (COX-1), has led to the important therapeutic development of COX-2 inhibitors."

Aspirin is a Cox-1 and traditional NSAIDs are both Cox-1 and Cox-2. Cox-1 is what can damage the lining of the stomach and lead to ulcers. Cox-2's have the safety of not interfering with gastric mucosal prostaglandin synthesis while having the anti-inflammatory and pain benefit.

Because of this risk, the Cox-2 medications, which include Celebrex and Vioxx, became some of the fastest growing and largest selling medications in history. This was mostly due to their marketing as well as their timing in the changing healthcare system. Dr. John Abramson[3] described his dilemma with Cox-2's as a practicing physician in his book Overdo$ed America. Dr. Abramson explains the predicament he was in with one of his patients demanding a prescription for Celebrex to cure his tennis elbow only based on a friend's recommendation. Dr. Abramson tried to help his patient by giving him some exercises along with an inexpensive NSAID, both of which have been proven to work for his issue. Unfortunately, the patient made it very clear that either he left with a prescription for Celebrex or he would find another physician who would. Against his better judgment, Dr. Abramson wrote the prescription.

Dr. Abramson mentioned the changing healthcare system and how patients began looking at their medications by how much their co-pay would be. The American patient has become more dependent on prescriptions while increasing their expectations gained from them. Instead of working out, take a pill. Instead of eating healthy, take a pill. Having insurance, which pays for the majority of the cost of the prescription, only makes it more inviting.

The popularity of the Cox-2's caused their downfall. Celebrex was the first Cox-2 on the market, launching in the United States in 1998. The CLASS (Celecoxib Long-term Arthritis Safety Study) was conducted from September 1998 until March 2000. It was published in the September 13, 2000 issue of the *Journal of the American Medical Association* (JAMA)[4]. CLASS was a phase 4 post-approval study which was required by the FDA and had over 8,000 patients enrolled. The data gathered was for 6 months. The results showed that patients taking Celebrex had a lower incidence of symptomatic ulcers and ulcer complications compared to NSAIDs.

Although the CLASS reported the 6-month data, Dr. Abramson pointed out that the study was designed for 12 months. The study went through the full 12 months, but only the first six months made it into the paper. Although the data from months seven through twelve wasn't in the article, it was on the FDA website. Dr. Abramson pointed out that six of the seven patients with serious gastrointestinal complications that occurred were patients taking Celebrex during months seven through twelve of the study.

Vioxx became the second Cox-2 on the market in 1999, and the VIGOR (Vioxx Gastrointestinal Outcomes Research) study was published in the *New England Journal of Medicine*[5] in the November 23, 2000 issue. The VIGOR study showed that patients taking Vioxx had fewer ulcers and less gastrointestinal bleeding compared to patients taking naproxen. A problem with the investigation is in the reporting. It is later reported that instead of 17 heart attacks of patients taking Vioxx there were 20.

A memo showed the extra three deaths, and then the study was updated.

There was evidence that Cox-2's might be beneficial regarding colon polyps and colon cancer, which Merck wanted to research with their APPROVe (Adenomatous Polyp Prevention on Vioxx) study. The results of the study showed an increased risk of heart attacks and strokes in patients taking Vioxx. "Cardiovascular Events Associated with Rofecoxib in a Colorectal Adenoma Chemoprevention Trial" was reported in the *New England Journal of Medicine* [6]May 17, 2005 issue.

In September 2004 Merck pulled Vioxx from the market. By the time it was removed, 20 million patients had taken Vioxx. Merck eventually paid $5 billion in settlements for the heart attacks and strokes caused by their blockbuster medicine.

With these Cox-2 concerns, the FDA conducted a study on Celebrex to determine its safety. In 2018, the FDA looked at data from 24,000 patients with osteoarthritis and rheumatoid arthritis, with one third each taking Celebrex, naproxen, or ibuprofen. It was determined that there is no evidence that Celebrex poses any higher risk for heart attacks or stroke compared to naproxen or ibuprofen.[7]

With the history of the Cox-2's completed, I will explain why I shared it. Prevacid was the first PPI with the NSAID indication, which was a big deal. Cox-2's were a multi-billion dollar class of medication that was marketed exceptionally well; however, they didn't have studies that showed they were better at relieving pain compared to NSAIDs. The benefit was that they were meant to be safer regarding gastric ulcers.

Takeda launched Prevacid NapraPAC (PNP) in 2003 with two strengths of naproxen, 375mg, and 500mg. It consisted of pills from both Prevacid and naproxen, the same NSAID as Aleve. The doses of naproxen were either 375mg or 500mg while the treatment of Prevacid was always only 15mg. The marketing campaign for Prevacid NapraPAC was that Cox-2's don't have any studies that show they work better than naproxen, just that they cause fewer gastric ulcers. With Prevacid NapraPAC, patients can get the benefit of the FDA approved NSAID indication for protection while receiving pain relief medication, and at the same time getting the heartburn relief benefits of Prevacid.

An issue that we would use in promoting Prevacid NapraPAC is when patients would take baby aspirin for cardiovascular protection. Taking a baby aspirin is something so small that patients might forget, or just not think to mention to their physician. The problem is when the patient is on a Cox-2 to protect their stomach but then takes the baby aspirin for their heart. Remember back to what aspirin is? A Cox-1 - which is the part that can damage the stomach lining. It would be beneficial for a patient taking aspirin to use Prevacid NapraPAC instead of a Cox-2.

Prevacid NapraPAC was a failure! Doctor's didn't want to write it for the main reason that it was only 15mg of Prevacid. Prevacid had a 15mg and a 30mg dose. It was almost always written as 30mg except for pediatrics. I heard over and over again that they would write PNP if it contained the higher 30mg, but the FDA approved dose for risk reduction of NSAID associated ulcers was 15mg, so Takeda wasn't allowed to package it with 30mg. Fast forward to the promotion of Dexilant, there is the option to promote a higher and a lower dose, the higher dose is encouraged.

Our goal was to switch patients that were on Prevacid over to Dexilant. Since we were regularly calling on rheumatologists with Prevacid, we were instructed to call on them for Dexilant as well. Remember, Prevacid had indications that rheumatologists would prescribe for, Dexilant does not! As representatives, we were paid for every prescription of Dexilant a rheumatologist wrote, and Takeda provided lists ranking the rheumatologists in order of importance for Dexilant sales. In a letter from Shinji Honda, President, and CEO of Takeda Pharmaceuticals North

America, Inc., "Kapidex (Dexilant) is building on Takeda's established presence in the PPI market. For more than a year, Takeda has been refocusing promotion, sales and sampling efforts to Kapidex."

Unfortunately, this was another part of the story that did not go our way. Again, since we couldn't show the difference between 30mg and 60mg sales data, what indication the prescription was written for, or who the patient was due to HIPAA regulations, we were stopped by the strict interpretation of Rule 9(b). The ruling from the 4th Circuit Court of Appeals states:

The original unedited version is at the end of the chapter. I have edited the text to make it easier to read.

First, Relator alleges in the amended complaint that Takeda promoted Kapidex to rheumatologists, who do not treat the conditions for which Kapidex has been approved.7 According to Relator, when promoting Kapidex to rheumatologists, Takeda sales representatives equated Kapidex with Prevacid, even though Kapidex was not approved for 10 of the 13 indications for which Prevacid was approved, including the gastric conditions commonly suffered by rheumatology patients. Relator further alleges that Takeda sales representatives were instructed to promote Kapidex to rheumatologists without disclosing that the drug is not approved for the gastric condition often experienced by rheumatology patients.

These allegations concerning the promotion of Kapidex to rheumatologists fall far short of the pleading standards set forth in Rule 9(b) and in Iqbal. Fatal to the claim, Relator does not allege in the amended complaint that the targeted rheumatologists wrote any off-label prescriptions that were submitted to the government for payment, a critical omission in a case brought under the Act.8 (holding that a complaint does not meet the requirements of Rule 9 when the complaint did not "give notice to the defendant of false claims submitted by others for federal reimbursement of off-label uses, only of illegal practices in promotion of the drug"), overruled on other grounds by Allison Engine Co. v. United ex rel. Sanders. Accordingly, Relator has not plausibly alleged that Takeda caused rheumatologists to write Kapidex prescriptions for off-label uses that actually were presented to the government for payment.

7ACCORDING TO RELATOR, rheumatologists do not treat GERD or EE, the two indications for which Kapidex is approved. Rheumatology patients may use Prevacid for gastric protection, a need associated with long-term ingestion of anti-inflammatory drugs such as Advil. However, as discussed above, Kapidex is not approved for gastric protection.

8After filing the amended complaint, Relator submitted to the district court a supplemental affidavit with attachments, which allegedly showed that two rheumatologists in Relator's sales territory wrote Kapidex prescriptions during a particular month. However, Relator cannot cure pleading deficiencies in the amended complaint with later-filed supporting documentation. Explaining that "matters beyond the pleadings cannot be considered on a Rule 12(b)(6) motion. (That even if I had new data showing the real prescription information, it couldn't be used). Moreover, we agree with the district court's observation that, even if these allegations had been included in the amended complaint, "there is nothing that prevents a rheumatologist from prescribing Kapidex for an approved condition at an approved dosage," and there was no indication in the record of the prescriptions' dosage, the conditions for which they were written, or that the prescriptions were submitted to the government for reimbursement.

· · ·

THE FOLLOWING IS **the original unedited version**

FIRST, Relator alleges in the amended complaint that Takeda promoted Kapidex to rheumatologists, who do not treat the conditions for which Kapidex has been approved.7 According to Relator, when promoting Kapidex to rheumatologists, Takeda sales representatives equated Kapidex with Prevacid, even though Kapidex was not approved for 10 of the 13 indications for which Prevacid was approved, including the gastric conditions commonly suffered by rheumatology patients. Relator further alleges that Takeda sales representatives were instructed to promote Kapidex to rheumatologists without disclosing that the drug is not approved for the gastric condition often experienced by rheumatology patients.

These allegations concerning the promotion of Kapidex to rheumatologists fall far short of the pleading standards set forth in Rule 9(b) and in Iqbal. Fatal to the claim, Relator does not allege in the amended complaint that the targeted rheumatologists wrote any off-label prescriptions that were submitted to the government for payment, a critical omission in a case brought under the Act.8 See United States ex rel. Rost v. Pfizer, Inc., 507 F.3d 720, 733 (1st Cir. 2007) (holding that a complaint does not meet the requirements of Rule 9 when the complaint did not "give notice to [the defendant] of false claims submitted by others for federal reimbursement of off-label uses, only of illegal practices in promotion of the drug"), overruled on other grounds by Allison Engine Co. v. United ex rel. Sanders, 553 U.S. 662 (2008). Accordingly, Relator has not plausibly alleged that Takeda caused rheumatologists to write Kapidex prescriptions for off-label uses that actually were presented to the government for payment.

7ACCORDING TO RELATOR, rheumatologists do not treat GERD or

EE, the two indications for which Kapidex is approved. Rheuma-tology patients may use Prevacid for gastric protection, a need associated with long-term ingestion of anti-inflammatory drugs such as Advil. However, as discussed above, Kapidex is not approved for gastric protection.

8After filing the amended complaint, Relator submitted to the district court a supplemental affidavit with attachments, which allegedly showed that two rheumatologists in Relator's sales terri-tory wrote Kapidex prescriptions during a particular month. However, Relator cannot cure pleading deficiencies in the amended complaint with later-filed supporting documentation. See E.I. du Pont de Nemours & Co. v. Kolon Indus., 637 F.3d 435, 448-49 (4th Cir. 2011) (explaining that "matters beyond the plead-ings . . . cannot be considered on a Rule 12(b)(6) motion"); Sec'y of State for Defence v. Trimble Navigation Ltd., 484 F.3d 700, 705 (4th Cir. 2007) (stating the documents that may be considered in evaluating a Rule 12(b)(6) motion). Moreover, we agree with the district court's observation that, even if these allegations had been included in the amended complaint, "there is nothing that prevents a rheumatologist from prescribing Kapidex for an approved condition at an approved dosage," and there was no indication in the record of the prescriptions' dosage, the condi-tions for which they were written, or that the prescriptions were submitted to the government for reimbursement.

14

FILING WITH THE DEPARTMENT OF JUSTICE IN PHILADELPHIA, PA

None of this would have happened if my wife (at the time) and our friends from Georgetown Law School were not involved. By working the case ourselves, we saved hundreds of thousands of dollars, but we also were not experienced in *qui tam* lawsuits. I am not blaming anyone that worked on my case, but we had some unfortunate events along the way. We tried to do the right thing, and so we gambled, and we lost.

During the lawsuit, we were criticized for amending our complaint several times, but the thing that most frustrates me is that when we started the case, Takeda only provided us with sales data combining sales of both Dexilant 60mg and Dexilant 30mg together. After the case began, when it was too late to add in new information, Takeda started to provide the sales data breaking down the sales of 60mg and 30mg into separate columns. One of Takeda's defenses in the case was that there was no proof that the physicians wrote the 60mg dose in my territory. Before the data changed I received an email, which was part of the case, that stated over 93% of Dexilant prescriptions nationally, were for the 60mg dose. The court ruled that it isn't plausible that the 93%

data can be used to represent my territory and in order to have a case I need to have my data to prove it.

Another critical thing to remember is that the information was available; it was just too late to add it. We had no way of knowing if or when Takeda would change the reports otherwise we could have waited to file until we had clear data showing the difference. The national sales data had 93% at Dexilant 60mg, and after we began receiving the updated data, it showed that my territory was at 95% 60mg.

It was an incredible amount of work to prepare the case for filing with the DOJ. I was able to provide my lawyers with sales reports, emails, and training materials but I was just a sales representative with limited written information. Having been with the company for over six years at the time, I had a lot of knowledge on PPI's and the ethics and compliance of selling them. I was promoting Prevacid with its numerous indications since I started with Takeda and now they were trying to replace Prevacid with Dexilant to try to limit the loss of the $3 billion in Prevacid sales instead of losing it to the generic market.

Another issue that was part of the case but not as important was our promotion to rheumatologists. We promoted Prevacid to rheumatologists for the indication of NSAID associated ulcers, but Dexilant did not have that indication. In pharmaceutical sales, we are only allowed to promote our products if it has the indication in our package insert, which created a problem in our promotion to rheumatologists. Takeda wanted them to use Dexilant where they had previously used Prevacid.

The Law Office of Bell & Bell LLP is in Philadelphia, PA and run by James and Jennifer Bell, two of my closest friends. They are both Georgetown Law School graduates who were close classmates with my ex-wife.

We filed the case with the Department of Justice in the Eastern District of Pennsylvania in Philadelphia, PA because the EDPA had experience in pharmaceutical *qui tams* and to our surprise, they responded in a few weeks. The DOJ attorneys asked if we are willing to have the case transferred to the Eastern District of Virginia office since I lived in Northern Virginia at the time. We agreed because of the speed with which the DOJ responded to our filing and having government involvement in the case is a huge step forward. Hindsight is 20/20, but if we had stayed in the Eastern District of Pennsylvania, the result might have been entirely different.

The Eastern District of Pennsylvania is in the Federal 3rd Circuit, and the Eastern District of Virginia is in the Federal 4th Circuit. The case is based on federal law so it shouldn't matter, but as you will see, federal law is not the same throughout the country. The main reason the U.S. Supreme Court was going to take my case is because of the federal circuit court split with:

WHETHER RULE 9(b) requires that a complaint under the False Claims Act "allege with particularity that specific false claims actually were presented to the government for payment," as required by the Fourth, Sixth, Eighth, and Eleventh Circuits, or whether it is instead sufficient to allege the "particular details of" the "scheme to submit false claims" together with sufficient indicia that false claims were submitted, as held by the First, Fifth, Seventh, and Ninth Circuits.

15

WEARING A WIRE

P hoenix, Arizona
January 2010

WHEN I WAS INFORMED by Takeda that we would be having a three-day sales meeting in Phoenix, AZ in January, I notified the government. During our meeting at FBI Headquarters, they had asked me if I would be willing to wear a wire and I said I would. I was going to get that opportunity and an experience I will never forget.

A few weeks before the sales meeting I met with one of the FBI Special Agents and the FDA Special Agent at an FBI building in the Washington, D.C. suburbs of Virginia. We discussed the logistics of the meeting, and they had prepared several wired shirts for me to try on. They had asked my shirt size the week before and needed to make sure the meeting was business casual and that I would not be wearing a tie, since a tie would block the camera. They picked the button-down dress shirts up at Costco. The shirts were designed with a camera that looked like and took the place of the third button down from the top, the typical place for a shirt to be buttoned without wearing a tie. There were two microphones, one under each side of the collar, and the wires from the microphones and the camera ran along the inside of the shirt and into a pouch, the size of a deck of cards, sewn under my right armpit. I later asked if I could keep the shirts as a souvenir, but I wasn't allowed to.

The Special Agents made reservations at the hotel where the meeting was taking place and went out early to meet me there. There were the two Special Agents I was already working with, one from each the FBI and FDA and we were joined by another FBI Special Agent.

The Special Agents had a room which was just for the operation with a lot of technical equipment and computers. That is where we would meet several times a day for me to change into one of their shirts as well as to change the batteries in the recording device.

I mentioned that the Special Agents went out early to set up and prepare for my arrival. Phoenix we have a problem. My flight was delayed, and in the process, the airlines lost my luggage. Since this is the type of thing, a writer would add in to make the story more exciting I produced my lost luggage receipt at the end of the chapter.

The Special Agents knew when my flight was supposed to land and they were texting me to check on my status and to inform me what room to meet them in. Since I was in flight and could not get their texts or calls, they were concerned and called my attorney. I am not sure if they thought I changed my mind after they went through the effort and expense of setting everything up, but they were very anxious to reach me. By the time I landed they had figured out that my flight was delayed and I was still in the air as the reason for not responding. Once I landed and turned on my phone, I was able to let them know my situation.

The dress code at the Takeda sales meeting was business casual, but since it was January, I left Virginia in jeans and a sweatshirt with the intention of changing at the hotel. The problem was the airlines lost my luggage! A co-worker of mine was on the same flight and waited with me while dealing with my lost bag. Because of that, and the fact that there weren't any clothing stores nearby, I couldn't show up at the meeting in a new shirt while still wearing jeans. My bag was eventually dropped off at the hotel later that night, but for the afternoon meeting, the Special Agents and I had to improvise.

I eventually made it to the meeting room, and since I couldn't change into one of their shirts, we decided just to record audio for the rest of the day. The unique shirts had a pouch sewn into them to hold the device, but since I was wearing my own clothes, the device was taped to my side, just like in the movies. With the device, that was the size of a deck of cards, taped to my right side, the wires and microphone needed to get to a spot for maximum ability without being seen. They had to cut my t-shirt to pass the wire through, and I had to be aware of making sure no one could see the shape of the box under my arm.

The audio worked fine, and there wasn't much going on in that afternoon meeting or dinner. After dinner, I went back to the meeting room and had the agents remove the device before going back to my own room, where I had a roommate.

The next morning I got dressed, and while my roommate was in the shower, I left and went one floor down to the Agent meeting room, which was just across the hall from the stairwell. My concern was that someone I knew from Takeda might see me going into that room. What if they thought it was my room and knocked on the door? Once inside the agents would give me the designed shirt with the special pocket and wires leading to the camera that was the button on my sternum and the microphones under both sides of my collar. The system recorded into the box, but they had to wait until they got it back to view it. They gave me an extra device so they could listen live, but it didn't work due to the distance and interference of the hotel.

At big meetings like this, you see people you have known for years that are scattered across the country, a lot of hugs are involved. If I were standoffish, it would have seemed odd, so I had to be concerned that someone would feel the hard drive under my right armpit. I am right handed, and I would keep my bicep over the rectangular box pinching it so it couldn't be felt. While it was in the pouch, sewn into the shirt, I was concerned that the corner of the box could be seen from behind and someone would ask about it. Along with losing the luggage for dramatic effect, I had a second issue arise the morning of the first full day of the meeting. All of us filed into a room for a presentation, and they had us sitting in rows of chairs. As we filed in, we walked down the rows filling in empty seats then beginning the next row of chairs. I was about to take my seat when I noticed my old manager ended up directly behind me! In the exact place thirty inches away from the rectangular box with the corners hanging under my right armpit. Of course, the chairs were short backed so I couldn't rely on the chair to block any edge that could be seen. I kept my right arm tight on my body to make sure the box was hidden and couldn't wait for that session to end.

That afternoon we were in a room working at round tables and having to write out different plans and scenarios as the task. Again, I am right handed, and I was afraid a corner of the box would show, so I had to write while trying to keep my arm as close to my body as possible. Needless to say, it was a challenging day, but one amusing thing I want you to think about is that once the camera and recording have started, the only reason it can be paused or turned off is by the FBI and FDA agents when they change out the battery. The first minute and the last minute of the recording has me reading a statement of my name and the date and time. They do this so they can't be accused of picking and choosing what to record or any issues like the missing Watergate tapes. I will say the first time I had to use the restroom that day was an experience. I am a big coffee drinker, so it was only the first of many visits where the FBI and FDA agents had to endure viewing urinals, but I did wash my hands.

After the meetings were over on the first full day, I went back to the agent's room for them to change out the battery in case there was anything worthwhile at the evening activities. I later went back to the room around 10pm, and they took off my unique shirt, and I changed back into the shirt I left my room wearing at 7:15 that morning.

The next morning at 7:15 I left my room while my roommate was in the shower, went down the stairs, and again crossed the hallway to the agent's room hoping no one would notice me. I told the agents that the pocket to hold the box was an issue, and we decided to tape it to my side like we did the first day. What a relief, it was very stressful worrying about someone seeing a pronounced corner of the unit and having to explain it. I still kept my right arm down as much as possible but a lot less stress.

A few hours into the day I received a text from the agents that they are watching the video from the previous day and the button camera was aiming high instead of straight ahead. To help, I started leaning down and moving my entire torso to record whoever was speaking or asking questions. I'm sure I looked a little odd but not enough to draw attention to myself.

I only ever saw a few seconds of the video, while I was having the batteries changed out in the afternoon on the second full day. The agents never discussed the recordings with me after the fact. I was not allowed to speak or acknowledge them outside of the room, but I would see them in the lobby, and one of the FBI agents was on my flight back home. I saw her showing the airline employee her documentation and her firearm, and although we didn't speak, we gave each other a nod of the head.

It definitely was an experience that I will never forget. I wasn't able to tell my friends that I worked with, but there wasn't anything negative that they needed to be concerned about. I kept the three white t-shirts that had cuts in them, to pass the wires through, and continued to wear them as regular undershirts for work. When I would grab a t-shirt from the drawer, and if it was one with a cut, I would always get a grin on my face thinking of the experience. I have since stopped wearing them and keep them as souvenirs.

UNITED

Delayed Baggage Report

A Delayed Baggage Report has been created for 1 bag.
You can check the status of your report online by visiting
www.united.com/bagtrack and entering the following information.

Report Number: M9H3Q2
Last Name: NATHAN
Claim Check Number: UA202181

If you do not have internet access and require additional assistance,
please call 1-800-221-6903. Please retain your claim check until your
baggage is delivered. In the unlikely event that your baggage is not
recovered, this may be required for claim settlement.

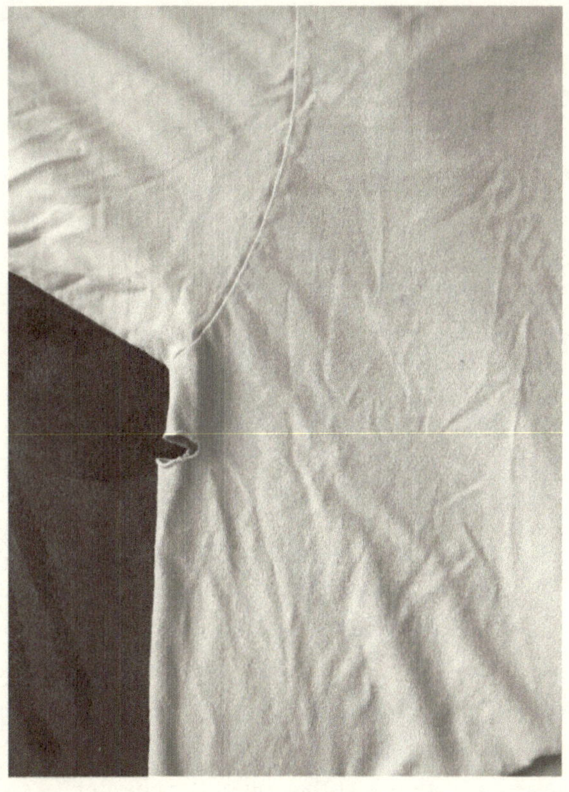

16

THE EASTERN DISTRICT OF VIRGINIA

The Eastern District of Virginia (EDVA) in Alexandria, VA. The EDVA is a Federal District Court in the 4th Circuit Court of Appeals system. Federal judges are nominated by the President of the United States and once approved by the Senate, are appointed for life.

The court's decision is at the end of the chapter.

The judge in my case was Anthony J. Trenga. Judge Trenga was nominated by President George W. Bush and was appointed to the bench in October 2008.[1]

In his decision, Judge Trenga stated:

"IT MAY WELL BE that doctors who prescribed a drug for off-label uses as a result of the defendant's illegal marketing of the drug withstood the temptation and did not seek federal reimbursement, and neither did their patients. It may be that physicians prescribed the drug for off-label uses only where the patients paid for it themselves, or when the patients' private insurers paid for it". As a result, Relator has failed to identify any false claims, or plead facts that would establish "beyond possibility" that false claims were in fact submitted, and Relator's Section 3729(a)(1)(A) claim will be dismissed for failure to state a claim.

THIS PREVIOUS PARAGRAPH from Judge Trenga's decision mentions the possibility of patients having insurance but instead of only paying their 20 percent co-pay (or other discounted rate) they decided to pay full price for their medicine. The patient, "withstood the temptation" to have their medication cost reimbursed.

To JUMP AHEAD, the Federal 4th Circuit Court of Appeals will use the same argument to not allow testimony from three physicians involved as expert witnesses in my case:

"IT MAY BE that physicians prescribed the drug for off-label uses only where the patients paid for it themselves or when the patients' private insurers paid for it." We therefore disagree with Relator's assertion that, if a patient is insured under a government program, we reasonably may infer that any prescription the patient received for an off-label use was filled and that a claim was presented to the government. For these reasons, we conclude that Relator's allegations in the amended complaint relating to the three physician affidavits do not adequately state that any false claims were presented to the government for payment.

In 2009, the United States Congress added an amendment to the False Claims Act. On May 20, 2009 the Fraud Enforcement and Recovery Act (FERA) of 2009 was signed into law by President Obama. The FERA was in response to a U.S. Supreme Court decision in Allison Engine Co. v. United States ex rel. Sanders.

Jeremy E. Gersh states in, "Saying What They Mean: The

False Claims Act Amendments in the Wake of Allison Engine"[2], Congress did not agree with the Supreme Court's decision in taking a restrictive approach to the FCA, and passed the amendment to clarify the law which the court will interpret in the future. "FERA completely rewrote § 3729 to return the statute to Congress's original intent. First, Congress rewrote § 3729(a)(2) by removing the phrase "paid or approved by the Government," and focused on "a false or fraudulent claim." Further, Congress added a materiality requirement to the FCA, defining materiality as "having a natural tendency to influence, or be capable of influencing, the payment or receipt of money or property." Now, a false statement only needs to be "material to a false or fraudulent claim," and there is no element of intent."

My legal documents to the EDVA contained:

60. Moreover, over the last decade, the scope of the False Claims Act ("FCA") has been broadened considerably by the adoption of the Fraud Enforcement and Recovery Act of 2009 ("FERA"), reflecting the clear intention of Congress to expand the reach of the FCA.

61. Indeed, FERA made clear that "intent' to submit a false claim is irrelevant, and that liability attaches even if an innocent third party submitted the actual false claim (e.g. physicians, pharmacists or patients).

MY LAWYERS ARGUED the district court misconstrued the relevant pleading standards under Federal Rules of Civil Procedure 12(b)(6) and 9(b). Under Rule 12(b)(6), a complaint must allege sufficient factual matter to state a plausible claim for relief.

. . .

TAKEDA'S BRIEF to the EDVA stated that they should prevail because:

NATHAN DOES NOT IDENTIFY a single doctor who was induced by a Takeda sales representative to write an off-label prescription for Kapidex. In fact, Relator does not identify a single doctor who has ever written an off-label prescription for Kapidex.

THEIR STATEMENT that I do not identify a single doctor is incorrect, my Complaint states:

AS SET FORTH HEREIN, several physicians, including Dr. Richard Corlin, a board-certified gastroenterologist and the former president of the American Medical Association, have attested, that Takeda's illegal promotion of Kapidex induced them to write 60 mg prescriptions of Kapidex for GERD. Indeed, these physicians have attested that they did not know that 60 mg Kapidex was not indicated for GERD and that they were not aware of a 30 mg Kapidex dose at all.

Dr. Bedford is a renowned endoscopist in the West Los Angeles medical community. Dr. Bedford completed his Internal Medicine internship and residency at the New York Hospital Cornell Medical Center and Memorial Sloan-Kettering Cancer Center in New York, NY, and he completed his gastroenterology fellowship at the Cleveland Fellowship program.

Until Drs. Corlin and Bedford were contacted by Relator's counsel in connection with this case, they were unaware that Kapidex was available in a 30 mg dosage form and that Kapidex 60 mg was not indicated for non-erosive GERD. Through their affidavits attached hereto, Drs. Corlin and Bedford have attested to the following:

(a) doctors are unlikely to write new prescriptions for PPIs, including Kapidex, unless a sample is available;

(b) doctors writing new prescriptions for PPI's, including Kapidex, typically conduct a "PPI trial," in which they provide a sample of a PPI to a patient, along with a prescription to fill if the patient has a positive experience with taking the samples;

(c) sampling influences doctors prescribing of PPIs, including Kapidex, and the exclusive availability of samples in a certain dosage makes it much more likely that a doctor would write a prescription at the sampled dosage, rather than another dosage;

(d) Takeda's exclusive sampling of Kapidex at 60 mg is likely to influence doctors to write more prescriptions at 60 mg than they otherwise would, because of the practice of conducting PPI trials, and because the exclusive sampling at 60 mg suggests to doctors that 60 mg is the only dosage available;

(e) Kapidex is no different than the PPI market generally in that the majority of Kapidex prescriptions are written to treat GERD (not erosive esophagitis);

(f) erosive esophagitis is diagnosed by gastroenterologists, who conduct endoscopies;

(g) Primary care physicians, ENTs and rheumatologists do not generally conduct endoscopies and do not diagnose EE;

(h) The fact that 93% of Kapidex scripts are being written at 60 mg is not proof that 60 mg is medically indicated for GERD, but instead a function of the market created by Takeda, especially by their sampling practices;

(i) medical literature does not support the use of 60 mg Kapidex for GERD;

(j) the class-wide labeling change made by the FDA in May 2010 states that patients should use the lowest dose of PPIs appropriate to the condition being treated, including Kapidex, to avoid safety risks, and Takeda's attempts to influence doctors to write 60 mg Kapidex for conditions that should be treated with 30 mg is inconsistent with this directive;

(k) statistics indicating that doctors often do not know the limitations of the indications for medicines they are writing prescriptions for are equally applicable in the context of PPIs -- especially for Kapidex which is a relatively new drug;

(l) doctors do not regularly read the package inserts for drugs;

(m) their [Dr. Corlin and Bedford's] office received Kapidex samples from Takeda sales representatives;

(n) they are more likely to prescribe a PPI if they have a sample, so that they can allow a patient to try it out for tolerance and symptom relief before filling a prescription;

(o) because of Takeda's marketing of 60 mg Kapidex, including the exclusive sampling of 60 mg Kapidex, they were not aware Kapidex had a 30 mg dose;

(p) they have prescribed Kapidex in 60 mg dose for GERD patients;

(q) their decision to prescribe 60 mg rather than 30 mg for GERD patients was significantly influenced by the fact that Takeda does not sample 30 mg; and some of the individuals that they prescribed 60 mg Kapidex to for GERD were over 65 years of age and were Medicare participants.

DR. MICHAEL E. YAFFE, M.D. is a board-certified physician practicing internal medicine in Columbus, OH. Until Dr. Yaffe was contacted by Relator's counsel in connection with this case, he was unaware that Kapidex was available in a 30 mg dosage form. Through his affidavit attached hereto, Dr. Yaffe has attested to the following:

(a) he is a primary care physician who treats patients for GERD and has received Kapidex samples from Takeda sales representatives;

(b) he does not conduct endoscopies and therefore, does not diagnose EE;

(c) doctors writing new prescriptions for PPI's, including

Kapidex, typically conduct a "PPI trial," in which they provide a sample of a PPI to a patient, along with a prescription to fill if the patient has a positive experience with taking the samples;

(d) sampling influences doctors prescribing of PPIs, including Kapidex, and the exclusive availability of samples in a certain dosage would make it much more likely that a doctor would write a prescription at the sampled dosage, rather than another dosage;

(e) Takeda's exclusive sampling of Kapidex at 60 mg is likely to influence doctors to write more prescriptions at 60 mg than they otherwise would have, because of the practice of conducting PPI trials, and because the exclusive sampling at 60 mg suggests to doctors that 60 mg is the only dosage available;

(f) Dr. Yaffe is more likely to prescribe a PPI if he has a sample, so that he can allow a patient to try the PPI out for tolerance and symptom relief before filling a prescription;

(g) because of Takeda's marketing of 60 mg Kapidex, including the exclusive sampling of 60 mg Kapidex, Dr. Yaffe was not aware Kapidex had a 30 mg dose;

(h) he has prescribed Kapidex in the 60 mg dose for GERD patients;

(i) his decision to prescribe 60 mg rather than 30 mg for GERD patients was significantly influenced by the fact that Takeda does not sample 30 mg; and

(j) some of the individuals that he prescribed 60 mg Kapidex to for GERD were over 65 years of age and were Medicare participants.

I JUST PROVIDED information from three physicians that have provided affidavits about their experience with Kapidex and their interactions with Takeda representatives. Dr. Corlin wasn't aware of a 30mg dose until after we reached out to him about being an expert witness. The next time his Takeda representative came to his office he asked about the 30mg dose and the representative told him there isn't one.

So, just to recap, Takeda states that, "Nathan does not identify a single doctor who was induced by a Takeda sales representative to write an off-label prescription for Kapidex. In fact, Relator does not identify a single doctor who has ever written an off-label prescription for Kapidex." I just showed 3 physicians that stated under oath that they were induced by Takeda sales representatives to write Kapidex 60mg for GERD, off-label since the 60mg is only indicated for Erosive Esophagitis.

THE NEXT POINT from Takeda's brief is:

THE COMPLAINT simply makes the conclusory allegation that "as a result of the acts of Defendants," the government paid for off-label Kapidex prescriptions. (SAC ¶ 105.) In doing so, the Complaint does not identify any claims for reimbursement of Kapidex prescriptions that were submitted to the government.

MY COMPLAINT HAD 98 claims for reimbursement of Kapidex prescriptions that were submitted to the government. I may have beaten this point to death but at that time our sales data was not broken down by 30mg and 60mg but I did have it, in writing, that 93% of Kapidex prescriptions were for the 60mg dose. My Complaint showed 98 prescriptions that were submitted to Medicare Part D from 16 Primary Care physicians which would not have a reason to prescribe 60mg for Erosive Esophagitis. These same physicians are described in Chapter 1. Proof! with their prescribing data revealed.

· · ·

<u>THE COURTS DECISION</u> **(edited)**

To make it easier to read I will clean it up for the general public while having the entire decision with cites at the end of the chapter.

UNITED STATES EX **Noah Nathan v. Takeda Pharmaceuticals North America, Inc.**

Case No. 1:09-cv-1086 (AJT) (E.D. Va. Sep. 6, 2011)

<u>MEMORANDUM OPINION</u>

In this False Claims Act case, the plaintiff, relator Noah Nathan ("Relator" or plaintiff) alleges that defendants Takeda Pharmaceuticals North America, Inc. and Takeda Pharmaceuticals America, Inc. (collectively "Takeda") engaged in a fraudulent marketing scheme that caused false claims to be filed with the United States, namely, requests for payment or reimbursement under the federal Medicare, Medicaid, TRICARE, CHAMPVA and Federal Employee Health Benefit programs, for "off-label" prescriptions of Takeda's drug Kapidex. By Order dated May 4, 2011, the Court dismissed Relator's Second Amended Complaint, with leave to amend, primarily on the grounds that Relator failed to plead facts with sufficient specificity to state a claim. On May 18, 2011, Relator filed a Third Amended Complaint; and on June 9, 2011, Takeda filed a Motion to Dismiss Relator's Third Amended Complaint (the "Motion") pursuant Fed. R. Civ. P. 12(b)(6) and Fed. R. Civ. P. 9(b).

Relator's Third Amended Complaint, like his Second Amended Complaint, fails to identify any specific false claims or any specific prescriptions, physicians, pharmacies, payments or reimbursements that caused such a false claim to be filed. (acknowledging failure to plead that specific off-label prescriptions were submitted for reimbursement by the government). Nevertheless, Relator opposes the Motion essentially on the grounds that he may satisfy the specificity requirements for fraud-based claims, such as those under the False Claims Act, by pleading statistics concerning the make-up of Kapidex sales, together with other allegations concerning Takeda's marketing campaign, the misrepresentations to prescribing physicians by Takeda sales representatives that were an integral part of that marketing strategy, the patient populations served by medical specialists to whom Takeda distributed sample 60 milligram dosages of Kapidex, and the medical conditions for which, and dosages at which, Kapidex is approved by the Food and Drug Administration (the "FDA"). Upon consideration of the Motion, the memoranda and exhibits in support thereof and in opposition thereto, and the arguments of counsel at a hearing on July 8, 2011, and for the reasons contained in this Memorandum Opinion, the Court finds that the Third Amended Complaint fails to state a claim on which relief may be granted and the Court will grant the Motion.

I. <u>BACKGROUND</u>

Although considerably more detailed, Relator's 126 page, 660 paragraph Third Amended Complaint, viewed in the light most favorable to Relator, is substantially the same in substance as Relator's Second Amended Complaint, which this Court dismissed by Order dated May 4, 2011. In sum, Relator contends that Takeda is illegally promoting Kapidex, a drug which is considered to be in the medical category of drugs known as proton pump inhibitors. Specifically, Relator alleges that Takeda has caused the filing of false claims, and made and used false statements that were material to false claims, by: (1) promoting Kapidex to rheumatologists, whose patients suffer from conditions for which Kapidex has not been approved for treatment; (2) misrepresenting, through its sales representatives, the nature and efficacy of Kapidex and how it compares with Takeda's Prevacid, a predecessor drug which had been approved for certain medical conditions for which Kapidex is not approved; and (3) exclusively providing 60 milligram sample doses to gastroenterologists, rheumatologists, otolaryngologists and primary care physicians, despite the fact that the great majority of these doctors' patients have conditions for which there is no approved dosage of Kapidex or for which the only approved dosage of Kapidex is 30 milligrams. As in the Second Amended Complaint, the Relator's Third Amended Complaint asserts claims pursuant to the FCA, and various state statutes. Relator seeks injunctive relief, treble damages, civil penalties, and attorney fees, costs and expenses.

II. ANALYSIS

A. Relevant Pleading Standard

Relator's Third Amended Complaint must satisfy both Fed. R. Civ. P. 12(b)(6) and 9(b). To satisfy Fed. R. Civ. P. 12(b)(6), "a complaint must contain sufficient factual matter, accepted as true, to 'state a claim to relief that is plausible on its face.'" "A pleading that offers labels and conclusions or a formulaic recitation of the elements of a cause of action will not do." Relator's FCA claim must also be pleaded with particularity pursuant to Rule 9(b). Rule 9(b) requires Relator to plead, with specificity, the "who, what, when, where, and how of the alleged fraud." ("an FCA plaintiff must, at a minimum, describe the time, place, and contents of the false representations, as well as the identity of the person making the misrepresentation and what he obtained thereby")

This Circuit adheres to a strict application of Rule 9(b) to FCA claims and both trial and appellate courts have repeatedly emphasized that Rule 9(b)'s particularity requirement must be satisfied in FCA cases. (affirming dismissal of FCA case in which the plaintiff "submitted only one invoice ... and failed to allege with particularity any alleged rebate or credit" that was not reported to the government, and rejecting argument that plaintiff should be excused from pleading with specificity because requisite information is in possession of defendants); (dismissing complaint because it did "not describe even a single instance in which a physician was influenced to prescribe the drug based on the defendant's misrepresentations, and where a claim was made by the pharmacist to the government"); (granting motion to dismiss, and explaining "a plaintiff's conclusion that fraudulent claims were submitted must be supported by particularized allegations regarding not only time, place and content, but also the identity of the person making the misstatement and what was obtained thereby"). There have been cases in this Circuit, relied on by the Relator, that have not required at the pleadings stage the identification of specific false claims, but only where there has been an adequate description of a fraudulent scheme that makes the submission of all claims for reimbursement submitted by the defendant fraudulent.

In advancing his claims, Relator relies on a less demanding standard, adopted by some courts outside this Circuit, that would permit Relator to proceed without alleging the "who. what, when, where, and how" as to specific claims submitted to the government in violation of the FCA as long as his complaint contains "factual or statistical evidence to strengthen the inference of fraud beyond possibility." However, courts in this Circuit have clearly explained that a relator's allegation that "fraud must be occurring" is not sufficient to satisfy Rule 9(b), and for the reasons discussed below, Relator's statistics-based version of this theory does not satisfy his obligation to plead his claims under the FCA with specificity.

B. Relator's Claim Pursuant to 31 U.S.C. § 3729(a)(1)(A) (Count I)

The FCA creates a cause of action against any person who "knowingly presents, or causes to be presented, a false or fraudulent claim for payment or approval." Relator's Third Amended Complaint, like his Second Amended Complaint, fails to plead facts sufficient to establish that any specific false claims were presented to the United States for payment or approval, or that Takeda's promotional activities caused such presentment.

1. <u>Presentment of a False or Fraudulent Claim for Payment or Approval</u>

Relator has failed to identify any specific instances in which Takeda caused a pharmacist or other healthcare provider to submit a claim for reimbursement to the government based on a non-reimbursable prescription. Nevertheless, Relator seeks to satisfy its pleading obligations through a combination of statistics and general allegations concerning the patient populations served by medical specialists to whom Kapidex was marketed, and to whom samples of Kapidex were distributed.

Relator first alleges that rheumatologists do not treat any conditions for which Kapidex has been approved, and therefore all prescriptions written by rheumatologists for Kapidex are off-label. Then, relying on an attached affidavit, rather than allegations actually made in the Third Amended Complaint (which only contends that Takeda engaged in a campaign to promote Kapidex to rheumatologists, Relator contends that rheumatologists in Relator's territory wrote two prescriptions during a sample month, July 2009, and that Relator's territory is one of over 500 territories in the United States. Based on these allegations, Relators contends that the two prescriptions must have been non-reimbursable under any government program and that there are "likely tens of thousands of prescriptions written by rheumatologists when all of the territories are accounted for during the 28 month period during which Kapidex has been promoted." . Completing the journey he must travel, the Relator then contends that "there should be no question that some of these prescriptions were reimbursed by government programs, given the other data presented by Relator indicating that a significant percentage of prescriptions from his territory and his district were submitted for reimbursement to government programs."

These allegations are insufficient to establish for the purposes of the FCA either that non-reimbursable prescriptions were written or, if they were non-reimbursable, that they were submitted for reimbursement. There is nothing about these allegations that establishes beyond a possibility that "tens of thousands of prescriptions" of Kapidex were written by rheumatologists and that "some of these prescriptions were reimbursed by government programs." In fact, even as to the two postulated prescriptions, there is no allegation that either was in fact submitted for reimbursement by a federal agency. Even if they were, there is nothing that prevents a rheumatologist from prescribing Kapidex for an approved condition at an approved dosage and Relator makes no allegations, either in or outside of his Third Amended Complaint, as to what these two prescriptions were for or for what dosage they were written. In short, these allegations are insufficient to plead an FCA violation even as to the two alleged prescriptions; and they certainly are inadequate to establish any claim as to any other prescriptions. (endorsing view that sample sizes of between five and thirteen are "too small to have any predictive value").

As an initial matter, as this Court clearly explained in its prior Order, Relator may not avoid dismissal by attempting to plug holes in his complaint with supplemental affidavits. The Court has considered the substance of these affidavits in order to assess whether Relator should be granted further leave to amend his complaint.

Relator next points to 16 primary care physicians from his district who received 60 milligram samples from Takeda, and who wrote 98 prescriptions for Kapidex that were submitted to Medicare for reimbursement. Relator first alleges that primary care physicians do not treat conditions for which the 60 milligram dose is appropriate, thus presumably making all of the 60 milligram prescriptions by primary care physicians off-label. However, he does not allege that the prescriptions issued were in fact for 60 milligram doses. To cure this gap in proof, Relator argues that it is reasonable to infer that over 90% of these prescriptions were, in fact, issued at the 60 milligram dose because over 90% of Takeda's overall sales of Kapidex are at the 60 milligram dose. Relator does not, however, allege any basis on which to assume that the overall level of 60 milligram doses, as a percentage of overall Kapidex sales, corresponds to the prescriptions that were actually issued by these primary care physicians. There are also no factual allegations that would lead this Court to conclude that primary care physicians, generally, prescribed 60 milligram doses of Kapidex at levels that correspond to Takeda's overall rate of Kapidex sales.

Similarly, Relator contends that approximately 9,000 Kapidex prescriptions were submitted for federal reimbursement in two particular sales districts during periods in 2009 and 2010. Compl. Relator does not allege, however, the dosages of these prescriptions: and these statistics suffer from the same inadequacies as those pertaining to the 16 primary care physicians discussed above in that Relator does not explain the basis for his assumption that the overall 90% rate of 60 milligram doses can be attributed to these prescriptions as well. Moreover, these statistics do not identify the types of doctors issuing the prescriptions, the types of illnesses for which they issued the prescriptions at issue, or whether the doctors were subjected to Takeda's sample distribution practices.

Finally, Relator points to several physicians who attest in sworn declarations that they were not aware that Kapidex was available in a 30 milligram dosage, and whom Relator claims prescribed 60 milligram Kapidex doses to Medicare patients over the age of 65 for conditions for which the 60 milligram dosage of Kapidex was not approved by the FDA. By supplemental affidavit, one of these physicians further avers that certain of these patients contacted his office for prescription refills. However, there are no allegations or averments as to when the alleged prescriptions were issued, or that any claims for payment were actually submitted to Medicare in connection with these prescriptions. (explaining "it may well be that doctors who prescribed a drug for off-label uses as a result of the defendant's illegal marketing of the drug withstood the temptation and did not seek federal reimbursement, and neither did their patients. It may be that physicians prescribed the drug for off label uses only where the patients paid for it themselves, or when the patients' private insurers paid for it"). As a result, Relator has failed to identify any false claims, or plead facts that would establish "beyond possibility" that false claims were in fact submitted, and Relator's Section 3729(a)(1)(A) claim will be dismissed for failure to state a claim.

2. <u>Causation</u>

The Third Amended Complaint, like the Second Amended Complaint, also fails to plead facts sufficient to make plausible Relator's claim that Takeda "caused" any off-label prescriptions to be issued. Courts recognize that physicians are not unsophisticated lay persons and it is reasonable to assume that they are familiar with relevant medical literature. This is not to say that off-label promotion cases cannot be prosecuted under the FCA. However, off-label FCA cases generally involve allegations that the judgment of a physician was altered or affected by the defendant's fraudulent activities, which also typically involve improper payments, benefits or inducements, or misrepresentations. (involving kickbacks, misrepresenting studies, FDA approval and the efficacy of the drug, and presenting doctors with studies supporting off-label use); (involving kickbacks, providing false information to doctors regarding the safety and efficacy of the drug, and misrepresentations regarding credentials); (noting that the relator alleged that defendants hired ghostwriters to write and submit articles favorable to their drug in journals, but attributed the work to doctors and nurses); In re Pharmaceutical Industry Average Wholesale Price Litigation, (explaining that the relator alleged the defendant paid "cash bribes" to hospitals). As this Court noted in its May 4, 2011 Order, physicians are not prohibited from prescribing drugs for off-label uses, and Relator has not made any allegations regarding kickbacks or other improper incentives or attempts to distort otherwise objective medical literature. Moreover, the Court finds, for the reasons discussed below, that Relator has failed to allege facts that would support an actionable misrepresentation claim. Accordingly, this Court finds that Relator has not pleaded facts that would articulate a plausible theory of causation, and Relator's Section 3729(a)(1)(A) claim will be dismissed on this basis as well.

The Court notes that there appears to be a division among the courts regarding whether, to establish causation in fact, the Court must apply a "substantial factor" test or a "but for" causation test to claims under the FCA. The Court concludes that there is no need to determine whether the "but for" test or the "substantial factor" test applies since the Court concludes that Relator's allegations are insufficient under either test.

C. **Relator's Claim Pursuant to 31 U.S.C. S 3729(a)(1)(B) (Count II)**

The FCA also imposes liability on any person who "knowingly makes, uses, or causes to be made or used, a false record or statement material to a false or fraudulent claim." Relator's allegations regarding the existence of affirmative misrepresentations do not, however, meet Rule 9(b)'s requirements For example, Relator alleges that a certain identified Takeda sales manager stated during an October 2009 training session that she had only been promoting Kapidex to rheumatologists for NSAID gastric protection, which is not a medically accepted indication, but does not allege what she said to the physicians, when the alleged statements to physicians were made or where the statements were made, or identify the physicians to whom she made the representations. Likewise. Relator's allegations regarding "Sales Representative E" ("SRE") do not identify the practice or the physician with whom SRE communicated, or when in May 2011 the meeting took place. Furthermore, Relator has not alleged what these physicians did as a result of these marketing efforts, or that the alleged false statements were material to a claim for payment, or even that the recipient physician(s) issued any off-label prescriptions, much less that any such prescriptions were submitted for federal reimbursement. In the absence of any alleged misrepresentations that would satisfy the requirements of Rule 9(b), the Court will also dismiss Relator's Section 3729(a)(1)(B) claim.

Relator's other allegations are even less detailed. --------

D. Leave to Amend and Supplemental Jurisdiction

Given the previous opportunities which this Court has granted Relator to file an amended complaint and to address the deficiencies that this Court identified in its May 4, 2011 Order, the Court finds that granting Relator leave to file a further amended complaint would be futile. Accordingly, this Court will dismiss Relator's FCA claims without leave to file a further amended complaint. The Court declines to exercise supplemental jurisdiction over Relator's state law claims, which are hereby dismissed without prejudice.

CONCLUSION

For the above reasons, the Court concludes that in the absence of specific instances of false claims presented because of Takeda's conduct, and in the absence of any actionable misrepresentations, Relator fails to state a claim under the FCA. Relator's statistical and general allegations concerning what ailments are treated by what physicians, and the general nature of Takeda's promotional activities, do not supply the needed specificity under Rule 9(b), do not satisfy Iqbal and Twombly, and do not raise an inference of fraud beyond mere possibility. The Court will therefore grant Takeda's Motion, dismiss Relator's FCA claims (Counts I and II) without leave to amend, and dismiss Relator's remaining state law claims (Counts III through XXVIII) without prejudice.

An appropriate Order will issue.

Anthony J. Trenga

. . .

UNITED STATES DISTRICT Judge
   Alexandria, Virginia
   September 6, 2011

THE FOLLOWING version is the original

UNITED STATES EX Noah Nathan v. Takeda Pharmaceuticals North America, Inc.
   Case No. 1:09-cv-1086 (AJT) (E.D. Va. Sep. 6, 2011)

MEMORANDUM OPINION

In this False Claims Act case, the plaintiff, relator Noah Nathan ("Relator" or plaintiff) alleges that defendants Takeda Pharmaceuticals North America, Inc. and Takeda Pharmaceuticals America, Inc. (collectively "Takeda") engaged in a fraudulent marketing scheme that caused false claims to be filed with the United States, namely, requests for payment or reimbursement under the federal Medicare, Medicaid, TRICARE, CHAMPVA and Federal Employee Health Benefit programs, for "off-label" prescriptions of Takeda's drug Kapidex. By Order dated May 4, 2011, the Court dismissed Relator's Second Amended Complaint, with leave to amend, primarily on the grounds that Relator failed to plead facts with sufficient specificity to state a claim. On May 18, 2011, Relator filed a Third Amended Complaint; and on June 9, 2011, Takeda filed a Motion to Dismiss Relator's Third Amended Complaint [Doc. No. 76] (the "Motion") pursuant Fed. R. Civ. P. 12(b)(6) and Fed. R. Civ. P. 9(b).

Relator's Third Amended Complaint, like his Second Amended Complaint, fails to identify any specific false claims or any specific prescriptions, physicians, pharmacies, payments or reimbursements that caused such a false claim to be filed. See Relator's Opp., at 18 (acknowledging failure to plead that specific off-label prescriptions were submitted for reimbursement by the government). Nevertheless, Relator opposes the Motion essentially on the grounds that he may satisfy the specificity requirements for fraud-based claims, such as those under the False Claims Act, 31 U.S.C. § 3729 et seq. (the "FCA"), by pleading statistics concerning the make-up of Kapidex sales, together with other allegations concerning Takeda's marketing campaign, the misrepresentations to prescribing physicians by Takeda sales representatives that were an integral part of that marketing strategy, the patient populations served by medical specialists to whom Takeda distributed sample 60 milligram dosages of Kapidex, and the medical conditions for which, and dosages at which, Kapidex is approved by the Food and Drug Administration (the "FDA"). Upon consideration of the Motion, the memoranda and exhibits in support thereof and in opposition thereto, and the arguments of counsel at a hearing on July 8, 2011, and for the reasons contained in this Memorandum Opinion, the Court finds that the Third Amended Complaint fails to state a claim on which relief may be granted and the Court will grant the Motion.

I. BACKGROUND

Although considerably more detailed, Relator's 126 page, 660 paragraph Third Amended Complaint, viewed in the light most favorable to Relator, is substantially the same in substance as Relator's Second Amended Complaint, which this Court dismissed by Order dated May 4, 2011. In sum, Relator contends that Takeda is illegally promoting Kapidex, a drug which is considered to be in the medical category of drugs known as proton pump inhibitors. Specifically, Relator alleges that Takeda has caused the filing of false claims, and made and used false statements that were material to false claims, by: (1) promoting Kapidex to rheumatologists, whose patients suffer from conditions for which Kapidex has not been approved for treatment; (2)

misrepresenting, through its sales representatives, the nature and efficacy of Kapidex and how it compares with Takeda's Prevacid, a predecessor drug which had been approved for certain medical conditions for which Kapidex is not approved; and (3) exclusively providing 60 milligram sample doses to gastroenterologists, rheumatologists, otolaryngologists and primary care physicians, despite the fact that the great majority of these doctors' patients have conditions for which there is no approved dosage of Kapidex or for which the only approved dosage of Kapidex is 30 milligrams. See e.g. 3d Am. Compl., ¶¶ 6, 129-222. As in the Second Amended Complaint, the Relator's Third Amended Complaint asserts claims pursuant to the FCA (Counts I & II), and various state statutes (Counts III through XXVIII). Relator seeks injunctive relief, treble damages, civil penalties, and attorney fees, costs and expenses.

II. ANALYSIS

A. Relevant Pleading Standard

Relator's Third Amended Complaint must satisfy both Fed. R. Civ. P. 12(b)(6) and 9(b). To satisfy Fed. R. Civ. P. 12(b)(6), "a complaint must contain sufficient factual matter, accepted as true, to 'state a claim to relief that is plausible on its face.'" Ashcroft v. Iqbal, 129 S. Ct. 1937, 1949 (2009); Bell Atlantic Corp. v. Twombly, 550 U.S. 544, 570 (2007). "A pleading that offers labels and conclusions or a formulaic recitation of the elements of a cause of action will not do." Iqbal, 129 S. Ct. at 1949(internal quotation marks omitted). Relator's FCA claim must also be pleaded with particularity pursuant to Rule 9(b). Rule 9(b) requires Relator to plead, with specificity, the "who, what, when, where, and how of the alleged fraud." United States ex. rel. Wilson v. Kellogg Brown & Root, Inc., 525 F.3d 370,379 (4th Cir. 2008) ("an FCA plaintiff must, at a minimum, describe the time, place, and contents of the false representations, as well as the identity of the person making the misrepresentation and what he obtained thereby") (internal quotation marks omitted).

This Circuit adheres to a strict application of Rule 9(b) to FCA claims and both trial and appellate courts have repeatedly emphasized that Rule 9(b)'s particularity requirement must be satisfied in FCA cases. See e.g. Wilson, supra; United States ex rel. Elms v. Accenture LLP, 341 Fed. Appx. 869, 873 (4th Cir. 2009) (affirming dismissal of FCA case in which the plaintiff "submitted only one invoice ... and failed to allege with particularity any alleged rebate or credit" that was not reported to the government, and rejecting argument that plaintiff should be excused from pleading with specificity because requisite information is in possession of defendants); United States ex rel. Radcliffe v. Purdue Pharma L.P., 582 F. Supp. 2d 766, 784 (W.D. Va. 2008) (dismissing complaint because it did "not describe even a single instance in which a physician was influenced to prescribe [the drug] based on [the defendant's] misrepresentations, and where a claim was made by the pharmacist to the government"); United States ex rel. Martinez v. Virginia Urology Ctr., P.C., Case No. 3:09-cv-442, 2010 U.S. Dist. LEXIS 77078, at * 12-15 (E.D. Va. Jul. 29,2010) (granting motion to dismiss, and explaining "a plaintiff's conclusion that fraudulent claims were submitted must be supported by particularized allegations regarding not only time, place and content, but also the identity of the person making the misstatement and what was obtained thereby"). There have been cases in this Circuit, relied on by the Relator, that have not required at the pleadings stage the identification of specific false claims, but only where there has been an adequate description of a fraudulent scheme that makes the submission of all claims for reimbursement submitted by the defendant fraudulent. See e.g. United States ex rel. Decesare v. Americare in Home Nursing, 757 F. Supp. 2d 573, 583 (E.D. Va. 2010).

In advancing his claims, Relator relies on a less demanding standard, adopted by some courts outside this Circuit, that would permit Relator to proceed without alleging the "who. what, when, where, and how" as to specific claims submitted to the government in violation of the FCA as long as his complaint contains "factual or statistical evidence to strengthen the inference of fraud beyond possibility." See e.g. In re Pharmaceutical Industry Average Wholesale Price Litigation, 538 F. Supp. 2d 367, 390 (D. Mass. 2008) (quoting United States ex rel. Rost v. Pfizer, 507 F.3d 720, 733(1st Cir. 2007)). However, courts in this Circuit have clearly explained that a relator's allegation that "fraud must be occurring" is not sufficient to satisfy Rule 9(b), see Decesare, 757 F. Supp. 2d at 583 (applying Elms, 341 Fed. Appx. at 873); and for the reasons discussed below, Relator's statistics-based version of this theory does not satisfy his obligation to plead his claims under the FCA with specificity.

B. <u>Relator's Claim Pursuant to 31 U.S.C. § 3729(a)(1)(A)</u> <u>(Count I)</u>

The FCA creates a cause of action against any person who "knowingly presents, or causes to be presented, a false or fraudulent claim for payment or approval." 31 U.S.C. § 3729(a)(1)(A). Relator's Third Amended Complaint, like his Second Amended Complaint, fails to plead facts sufficient to establish that any specific false claims were presented to the United States for payment or approval, or that Takeda's promotional activities caused such presentment.

1. <u>Presentment of a False or Fraudulent Claim for Payment or</u> <u>Approval</u>

Relator has failed to identify any specific instances in which Takeda caused a pharmacist or other healthcare provider to submit a claim for reimbursement to the government based on a non-reimbursable prescription. Nevertheless, Relator seeks to satisfy its pleading obligations through a combination of statistics and general allegations concerning the patient populations served by medical specialists to whom Kapidex was marketed, and to whom samples of Kapidex were distributed.

Relator first alleges that rheumatologists do not treat any conditions for which Kapidex has been approved, and therefore all prescriptions written by rheumatologists for Kapidex are off-label. See e.g., 3d Am. Compl., ¶ 6. Then, relying on an attached affidavit, rather than allegations actually made in the Third Amended Complaint (which only contends that Takeda engaged in a campaign to promote Kapidex to rheumatologists, 3d Am. Compl., 149-169), Relator contends that rheumatologists in Relator's territory wrote two prescriptions during a sample month, July 2009, and that Relator's territory is one of over 500 territories in the United States. Based on these allegations, Relators contends that the two prescriptions must have been non-reimbursable under any government program and that there are "likely tens of thousands of prescriptions written by rheumatologists when all of the territories are accounted for during the 28 month period during which Kapidex has been promoted." Relator's Opp., at 13. Completing the journey he must travel, the Relator then contends that "there should be no question that some of these prescriptions were reimbursed by government programs, given the other data presented by Relator indicating that a significant percentage of prescriptions from his territory and his district were submitted for reimbursement to government programs." Id.

These allegations are insufficient to establish for the purposes of the FCA either that non-reimbursable prescriptions were written or, if they were non-reimbursable, that they were submitted for reimbursement. There is nothing about these allegations that establishes beyond a possibility that "tens of thousands of prescriptions" of Kapidex were written by rheumatologists and that "some of these prescriptions were reimbursed by government programs." In fact, even as to the two postulated prescriptions, there is no allegation that either was in fact submitted for reimbursement by a federal agency. Even if they were, there is nothing that prevents a rheumatologist from prescribing Kapidex for an approved condition at an approved dosage and Relator makes no allegations, either in or outside of his Third Amended Complaint, as to what these two prescriptions were for or for what dosage they were written. In short, these allegations are insufficient to plead an FCA violation even as to the two alleged prescriptions; and they certainly are inadequate to establish any claim as to any other prescriptions. See e.g. Birkbeck v. Marvel Lighting Corp., 30 F.3d 507, 511 (4th Cir. 1994) (endorsing view that sample sizes of between five and thirteen are "too small to have any predictive value").

As an initial matter, as this Court clearly explained in its prior Order, Relator may not avoid dismissal by attempting to plug holes in his complaint with supplemental affidavits. The Court has considered the substance of these affidavits in order to assess whether Relator should be granted further leave to amend his complaint.

Relator next points to 16 primary care physicians from his district who received 60 milligram samples from Takeda, and who wrote 98 prescriptions for Kapidex that were submitted to Medicare for reimbursement. Relator first alleges that primary care physicians do not treat conditions for which the 60 milligram dose is appropriate, thus presumably making all of the 60 milligram prescriptions by primary care physicians off-label. However, he does not allege that the prescriptions issued were in fact for 60 milligram doses. See 3d Am. Compl., ¶¶ 284-301. To cure this gap in proof, Relator argues that it is reasonable to infer that over 90% of these prescriptions were, in fact, issued at the 60 milligram dose because over 90% of Takeda's overall sales of Kapidex are at the 60 milligram dose. 3d Am. Compl., ¶¶ 310,345-348. Relator does not, however, allege any basis on which to assume that the overall level of 60 milligram doses, as a percentage of overall Kapidex sales, corresponds to the prescriptions that were actually issued by these primary care physicians. There are also no factual allegations that would lead this Court to conclude that primary care physicians, generally, prescribed 60 milligram doses of Kapidex at levels that correspond to Takeda's overall rate of Kapidex sales.

Similarly, Relator contends that approximately 9,000 Kapidex prescriptions were submitted for federal reimbursement in two particular sales districts during periods in 2009 and 2010. 3d Am. Compl., ¶¶ 312-313. Relator does not allege, however, the dosages of these prescriptions: and these statistics suffer from the same inadequacies as those pertaining to the 16 primary care physicians discussed above in that Relator does not explain the basis for his assumption that the overall 90% rate of 60 milligram doses can be attributed to these prescriptions as well. See 3d Am. Compl., ¶¶ 314, 345-348. Moreover, these statistics do not identify the types of doctors issuing the prescriptions, the types of illnesses for which they issued the prescriptions at issue, or whether the doctors were subjected to Takeda's sample distribution practices.

Finally, Relator points to several physicians who attest in sworn declarations that they were not aware that Kapidex was available in a 30 milligram dosage, and whom Relator claims prescribed 60 milligram Kapidex doses to Medicare patients over the age of 65 for conditions for which the 60 milligram dosage of Kapidex was not approved by the FDA 3d Am. Compl., ¶ 278, 281, Ex. 9, 10, 14. By supplemental affidavit, one of these physicians further avers that certain of these patients contacted his office for prescription refills. Yaffe Aff. [Doc. No. 81-3], at ¶ 3. However, there are no allegations or averments as to when the alleged prescriptions were issued, or that any claims for payment were actually submitted to Medicare in connection with these prescriptions. See e.g. Rost, 507 F.3d at 733(explaining "[i]t may well be that doctors who prescribed [a drug] for off-label uses as a result of [the defendant's] illegal marketing of the drug withstood the temptation and did not seek federal reimbursement, and neither did their patients. It may be that physicians prescribed [the drug] for off label uses only where the patients paid for it themselves, or when the patients' private insurers paid for it"). As a result, Relator has failed to identify any false claims, or plead facts that would establish "beyond possibility" that false claims were in fact submitted, and Relator's Section 3729(a)(1)(A) claim will be dismissed for failure to state a claim.

2. <u>Causation</u>

The Third Amended Complaint, like the Second Amended Complaint, also fails to plead facts sufficient to make plausible Relator's claim that Takeda "caused" any off-label prescriptions to be issued. Courts recognize that physicians are not unsophisticated lay persons and it is reasonable to assume that they are familiar with relevant medical literature. See United States ex rel. Polansky v. Pfizer, Inc., Case No. 04-cv-0704, 2009 U.S. Dist. LEXIS 43438, at * 19 (E.D.N.Y. May 22, 2009). This is not to say that off-label promotion cases cannot be prosecuted under the FCA. However, off-label FCA cases generally involve allegations that the judgment of a physician was altered or affected by the defendant's fraudulent activities, which also typically involve improper payments, benefits or inducements, or misrepresentations. See e.g. United States ex rel. Carpenter v. Abbott Labs, Inc., 723 F. Supp. 2d 395, 398-400 (D. Mass. 2010) (involving kickbacks, misrepresenting studies, FDA approval and the efficacy of the drug, and presenting doctors with studies supporting off-label use); United States ex rel. Franklin v. Parke-Davis, 147 F. Supp. 2d 39, 45-46 (D. Mass. 2001) (involving kickbacks, providing false information to doctors regarding the safety and efficacy of the drug, and misrepresentations regarding credentials); Strom ex rel. United States v. Scios. Inc., 676 F. Supp. 2d 884. 888-89 (N.D. Cal. 2009) (noting that the relator alleged that defendants hired ghost-writers to write and submit articles favorable to their drug in journals, but attributed the work to doctors and nurses); In re Pharmaceutical Industry Average Wholesale Price Litigation, 538 F. Supp. 2d at 37374 (explaining that the relator alleged the defendant paid "cash bribes" to hospitals). As this Court noted in its

May 4, 2011 Order, physicians are not prohibited from prescribing drugs for off-label uses, and Relator has not made any allegations regarding kickbacks or other improper incentives or attempts to distort otherwise objective medical literature. Moreover, the Court finds, for the reasons discussed below, that Relator has failed to allege facts that would support an actionable misrepresentation claim. Accordingly, this Court finds that Relator has not pleaded facts that would articulate a plausible theory of causation, and Relator's Section 3729(a)(1)(A) claim will be dismissed on this basis as well.

The Court notes that there appears to be a division among the courts regarding whether, to establish causation in fact, the Court must apply a "substantial factor" test or a "but for" causation test to claims under the FCA. See e.g., United States ex rel. Franklin Parke-Davis, Case No. 96-11651-PBS, 2003 U.S. Dist. LEXIS 15754, at * 12-13(D. Mass. 2003); United States ex rel. Hess v. Sanofi-Synthelabo Inc., Case No. 4:05CV570MLM, 2006 U.S. Dist. LEXIS 22449, at * 23 (E.D. Mo. Apr. 21, 2006). The Court concludes that there is no need to determine whether the "but for" test or the "substantial factor" test applies since the Court concludes that Relator's allegations are insufficient under either test.

C. Relator's Claim Pursuant to 31 U.S.C. S 3729(a)(1)(B) (Count II)

The FCA also imposes liability on any person who "knowingly makes, uses, or causes to be made or used, a false record or statement material to a false or fraudulent claim." 31 U.S.C. § 3729(a)(1)(B). Relator's allegations regarding the existence of affirmative misrepresentations do not, however, meet Rule 9(b)'s requirements For example, Relator alleges that a certain identified Takeda sales manager stated during an October 2009 training session that she had only been promoting Kapidex to rheumatologists for NSAID gastric protection, which is not a medically accepted indication, but does not allege what she said to the physicians, when the alleged statements to physicians were made or where the statements were made, or identify the physicians to whom she made the representations. 3d Am. Compl., ¶ 155. Likewise. Relator's allegations regarding "Sales Representative E" ("SRE") do not identify the practice or the physician with whom SRE communicated, or when in May 2011 the meeting took place. 3d Am. Compl., ¶ 251. Furthermore, Relator has not alleged what these physicians did as a result of these marketing efforts, or that the alleged false statements were material to a claim for payment, or even that the recipient physician(s) issued any off-label prescriptions, much less that any such prescriptions were submitted for federal reimbursement.In the absence of any alleged misrepresentations that would satisfy the requirements of Rule 9(b), the Court will also dismiss Relator's Section 3729(a)(1)(B) claim.

Relator's other allegations are even less detailed. See e.g. 3d Am. Compl., ¶¶ 232-250.

D. <u>Leave to Amend and Supplemental Jurisdiction</u>

Given the previous opportunities which this Court has granted Relator to file an amended complaint and to address the deficiencies that this Court identified in its May 4, 2011 Order, the Court finds that granting Relator leave to file a further amended complaint would be futile. Accordingly, this Court will dismiss Relator's FCA claims without leave to file a further amended complaint. The Court declines to exercise supplemental jurisdiction over Relator's state law claims (Counts III through XXVIII), which are hereby dismissed without prejudice.

<u>CONCLUSION</u>

For the above reasons, the Court concludes that in the absence of specific instances of false claims presented because of Takeda's conduct, and in the absence of any actionable misrepresentations, Relator fails to state a claim under the FCA. Relator's statistical and general allegations concerning what ailments are treated by what physicians, and the general nature of Takeda's promotional activities, do not supply the needed specificity under Rule 9(b), do not satisfy Iqbal and Twombly, and do not raise an inference of fraud beyond mere possibility. The Court will therefore grant Takeda's Motion, dismiss Relator's FCA claims (Counts I and II) without leave to amend, and dismiss Relator's remaining state law claims (Counts III through XXVIII) without prejudice.

An appropriate Order will issue.

Anthony J. Trenga

United States District Judge
Alexandria, Virginia
September 6, 2011

17

THE 4TH CIRCUIT COURT OF APPEALS

My appeal from the Eastern District of Virginia was heard by a three-judge panel in the 4th Circuit Court of Appeals in Richmond, VA.

For our appeal, we decided we needed proven experience and luckily our first choice accepted our case. MoloLamken, LLP is a very experienced appellate firm with brilliant attorneys. Our principal attorney was Jeff Lamken and his second chair was Mike Pattillo, Jr. They did an incredible job but unfortunately were fighting an uphill battle with the Eastern District of Virginia's ruling stating that the 4th circuit:

THIS CIRCUIT ADHERES to a strict application of Rule 9(b) to FCA claims and both trial, and appellate courts have repeatedly emphasized that Rule 9(b)'s particularity requirement must be satisfied in FCA cases.

WITH THE FACT that "this circuit adheres to a strict application of

Rule 9(b) to FCA claims" staring us in the face, made for an extremely uphill battle.

To EXCLUDE SWORN testimony from three physicians about their first-hand knowledge and experience, the ruling from the 4th circuit court of appeals contains:

"IT MAY BE that physicians prescribed the drug for off-label uses only where the patients paid for it themselves or when the patients' private insurers paid for it." We therefore disagree with Relator's assertion that, if a patient is insured under a government program, we reasonably may infer that any prescription the patient received for an off-label use was filled and that a claim was presented to the government. For these reasons, we conclude that Relator's allegations in the amended complaint relating to the three physician affidavits do not adequately state that any false claims were presented to the government for payment.

THE 4TH CIRCUIT COURT OF APPEALS agreed with the lower court that I "failed to plausibly allege that any false claims had been presented to the government for payment."

Since I could not provide the 60mg sales data during the legal process to win my case, I am showing it in this book to prove my case in the forum of public opinion.

THE COURT's **decision (edited)**

To make it easier to read I will clean it up for the general public while having the entire decision with cites at the end of the chapter.

. . .

UNITED STATES COURT OF APPEALS, FOURTH Circuit.

UNITED STATES ex rel. Noah NATHAN, On Behalf Of The United States Government and the States, Plaintiff–Appellant, v. TAKEDA PHARMACEUTICALS NORTH AMERICA, INCORPORATED; Takeda Pharmaceuticals America, Incorporated, Defendants–Appellees.

No. 11–2077.

Decided: January 11, 2013

Before MOTZ and KEENAN, Circuit Judges, and James K. BREDAR, United States District Judge for the District of Maryland, sitting by designation.ARGUED:Jeffrey A. Lamken, Mololamken, LLP, Washington, D.C., for Appellant. William F. Cavanaugh, Jr., Patterson, Belknap, Webb & Tyler, New York, New York, for Appellees. ON BRIEF:Michael G. Pattillo, Jr., Martin V. Totaro, Mololamken, LLP, Washington, D.C., for Appellant. Susan R. Podolsky, The Law Offices of Susan R. Podolsky, Alexandria, Virginia; Daniel S. Ruzumna, Sean H. Murray, Aileen M. McGill, Patterson, Belknap, Webb & Tyler, New York, New York, for Appellees.

OPINION

Noah Nathan (Relator), a sales manager for Takeda Pharmaceuticals (Takeda), brought this qui tam action against his employer under the False Claims Act (the Act). Relator alleges that Takeda violated the Act by causing false claims to be presented to the government for payment under Medicare and other federal health insurance programs. After allowing Relator to file a third amended complaint (the amended complaint), the district court dismissed Relator's claims under Federal Rule of Civil Procedure 12(b)(6). In this appeal, Relator argues that the district court erred in concluding that Relator did not plausibly allege in the amended complaint that false claims had been presented to the government for payment, or that Takeda caused the presentment of any such false claims. Relator also contends that the district court abused its discretion in denying Relator's request for leave to file a fourth amended complaint.

Upon our review, we hold that the district court did not err in dismissing the amended complaint, because Relator failed to plausibly allege that any false claims had been presented to the government for payment. We further hold that the district court did not abuse its discretion in denying Relator leave to file a fourth amended complaint.

I.

Among other things, the Act prohibits any person from knowingly "causing to be presented" to the government false claims for payment or approval. A false statement is actionable under the Act only if it constitutes a "false or fraudulent claim." Importantly, to trigger liability under the Act, a claim actually must have been submitted to the federal government for reimbursement, resulting in "a call upon the government fisc (treasury)."

Relator alleges in the amended complaint that prescriptions written for certain medical uses, which have not been approved by the Food and Drug Administration (the FDA) or included in statutorily specified compendia, are not reimbursable under federal health insurance programs. Such uses commonly are referred to as "off-label" uses. Relator further alleges that because the cost of prescriptions for off-label uses is not subject to reimbursement by the federal government, the presentment of these types of claims for payment constitutes a violation of the Act.

In the amended complaint, Relator additionally alleges that Takeda marketed its prescription drug Kapidex, a proton pump inhibitor used to treat various gastric conditions, for off-label uses. Relator alleges that two of Takeda's marketing practices caused presentation of false claims to the government. The identified marketing practices were: (1) Takeda's promotion of Kapidex to rheumatologists, who typically do not treat patients having conditions for which Kapidex has been approved; and (2) Takeda's practice of marketing high doses of Kapidex for the treatment of conditions for which only a lower dose has been approved by the FDA.

In particular, Relator alleges that 60 mg doses of Kapidex have been approved by the FDA only for the treatment of the active condition of erosive esophagitis (EE). However, Kapidex has been approved by the FDA at a lower 30 mg dose to treat the more common condition of gastroesophogeal reflux disease (GERD), as well as for the maintenance of already "healed" cases of EE. Relator alleges that Takeda has provided doctors with samples of Kapidex exclusively in 60 mg doses, irrespective whether such physicians treat active cases of EE. As Relator further alleges, by this sampling practice, Takeda improperly implies that a 60 mg dose of Kapidex is the only available dosage of that drug, thereby causing doctors to prescribe 60 mg doses for unapproved conditions. Relator also alleges that Takeda sales representatives regularly misled physicians by deflecting or dismissing their questions about proper dosages, and by making misrepresentations concerning the available dosages.

Additionally, Relator alleges that the motivation for Takeda's alleged fraudulent marketing stems from Takeda's desire to replicate the success of its previously approved drug, Prevacid, the patent for which was set to expire in 2009. Prevacid has been approved to treat 13 conditions, including GERD. Prevacid also has been approved to provide gastric protection and to treat gastric ulcers, indications relevant to rheumatology patients who regularly take anti-inflammatory pain medications. In contrast, Kapidex is not approved for these two conditions. Relator alleges that because the patent expiration date for Prevacid was approaching, Takeda promoted Kapidex to "fill the Prevacid void."

The district court dismissed the amended complaint on two independent grounds: (1) the amended complaint failed to allege the "presentment" of a false or fraudulent claim to the government for payment or approval; and (2) the amended complaint failed to allege adequately that Takeda "caused" the issuance of off-label prescriptions. The district court also denied Relator's request to amend his complaint for a fourth time. Because we conclude that the district court properly dismissed the amended complaint based on Relator's failure to allege presentment of a false claim, we do not reach the additional question whether Relator alleged sufficient facts to support the required causation element for a claim asserted under the Act. We further hold that the district court did not abuse its discretion in denying Relator's motion for leave to file a fourth amended complaint.

II.

We review de novo the district court's dismissal of a complaint for failure to state a claim. To survive a Rule 12(b)(6) motion to dismiss, a complaint must "state a claim to relief that is plausible on its face." Facts that are "merely consistent with" liability do not establish a plausible claim to relief. In addition, although we must view the facts alleged in the light most favorable to the plaintiff, we will not accept "legal conclusions couched as facts or unwarranted inferences, unreasonable conclusions, or arguments."

Before addressing the substantive allegations in the amended complaint, we first state the pleading requirements for fraud-based claims brought under the Act. In addition to meeting the plausibility standard of Iqbal, fraud claims under the Act must be pleaded with particularity pursuant to Rule 9(b) of the Federal Rules of Civil Procedure. Rule 9(b) provides:

In alleging fraud or mistake, a party must state with particularity the circumstances constituting fraud or mistake. Malice, intent, knowledge, and other conditions of a person's mind may be alleged generally.

To satisfy Rule 9(b), a plaintiff asserting a claim under the Act "must, at a minimum, describe the time, place, and contents of the false representations, as well as the identity of the person making the misrepresentation and what he obtained thereby."

The parties dispute the proper application of Rule 9(b) in this case. In Relator's view, to meet the requirements for pleading a fraud claim under the Act, a relator need only allege the existence of a fraudulent scheme that supports the inference that false claims were presented to the government for payment. In contrast, Takeda argues that Rule 9(b) requires that a relator plead facts plausibly alleging that particular, identifiable false claims actually were presented to the government for payment.

In view of the rationale underlying Rule 9(b), we decline to adopt Relator's argument for a more lenient application of the Rule. We have adhered firmly to the strictures of Rule 9(b) in applying its terms to cases brought under the Act. The multiple purposes of Rule 9(b), namely, of providing notice to a defendant of its alleged misconduct, of preventing frivolous suits, of "eliminating fraud actions in which all the facts are learned after discovery," and of "protecting defendants from harm to their goodwill and reputation," are as applicable in cases brought under the Act as they are in other fraud cases. Indeed, such purposes may apply with particular force in the context of the Act, given the potential consequences flowing from allegations of fraud by companies who transact business with the government. Moreover, we have emphasized that a claim brought under the Act that "rests primarily on facts learned through the costly process of discovery is precisely what Rule 9(b) seeks to prevent." For these reasons, nothing in the Act or in our customary application of Rule 9(b) suggests that a more relaxed pleading standard is appropriate in this case.

Neither are we persuaded by Relator's contention that allegations of a fraudulent scheme, in the absence of an assertion that a specific false claim was presented to the government for payment, is a sufficient basis on which to plead a claim under the Act in compliance with Rule 9(b). As the Supreme Court has cautioned, the Act "was not designed to punish every type of fraud committed upon the government." Instead, the critical question is whether the defendant caused a false claim to be presented to the government, because liability under the Act attaches only to a claim actually presented to the government for payment, not to the underlying fraudulent scheme. Therefore, when a relator fails to plead plausible allegations of presentment, the relator has not alleged all the elements of a claim under the Act. ("We cannot be left wondering whether a plaintiff has offered mere conjecture or a specifically pleaded allegation on an essential element of the lawsuit.").

We agree with the Eleventh Circuit's observation that the particularity requirement of Rule 9(b) "does not permit a False Claims Act plaintiff merely to describe a private scheme in detail but then to allege simply and without any stated reason for his belief that claims requesting illegal payments must have been submitted, were likely submitted or should have been submitted to the Government." Rather, Rule 9(b) requires that "some indicia of reliability" must be provided in the complaint to support the allegation that an actual false claim was presented to the government. Indeed, without such plausible allegations of presentment, a relator not only fails to meet the particularity requirement of Rule 9(b), but also does not satisfy the general plausibility standard of Iqbal. "If Rule 9(b) is to carry any water, it must mean that an essential allegation and circumstance of fraudulent conduct cannot be alleged in such conclusory fashion."; requiring relator to "provide some representative examples of the defendants' alleged fraudulent conduct".

Our conclusion is not altered by the cases cited by Relator, in which courts have held that the requirements of Rule 9(b) can be satisfied in the absence of particularized allegations of specific false claims. Based on the nature of the schemes alleged in many of those cases, specific allegations of the defendant's fraudulent conduct necessarily led to the plausible inference that false claims were presented to the government.

For example, in United States ex rel. Grubbs v. Kanneganti,

the relator alleged a conspiracy by doctors to seek reimbursement from governmental health programs for services that never were performed. The court concluded that, because the complaint included the dates of specific services that were recorded by the physicians but never were provided, such allegations constituted "more than probable, nigh (near in time) likely, circumstantial evidence that the doctors' fraudulent records caused the hospital's billing system in due course to present fraudulent claims to the Government." Accordingly, the court further concluded that it would "stretch the imagination" for the doctors to continually record services that were not provided, but "to deviate from the regular billing track at the last moment so that the recorded, but unprovided, services never get billed." (holding that, in scheme alleging kickbacks to health care providers, allegations regarding "the dates and amounts of the false claims filed by these providers with the Medicare program" met the standard imposed by Rule 9(b)).

Applying these principles, we hold that when a defendant's actions, as alleged and as reasonably inferred from the allegations, could have led, but need not necessarily have led, to the submission of false claims, a relator must allege with particularity that specific false claims actually were presented to the government for payment. To the extent that other cases apply a more relaxed construction of Rule 9(b) in such circumstances, we disagree with that approach.

In reaching this conclusion, we acknowledge the practical challenges that a relator may face in cases such as the present one, in which a relator may not have independent access to records such as prescription invoices, and where privacy laws may pose a barrier to obtaining such information without court involvement. Nevertheless, our pleading requirements do not permit a relator to bring an action without pleading facts that support all the elements of a claim. (noting "the basic pleading requirement that a plaintiff set forth facts sufficient to allege each element of his claim"). We further emphasize, however, that the standard we articulate today does not foreclose claims under the Act when a relator plausibly pleads that specific, identifiable claims actually were presented to the government for payment. Of course, whether such factual allegations in a given case meet the required standard must be evaluated on a case-specific basis.

III.

Employing the above pleading standard, we turn to consider the sufficiency of the amended complaint in this case. Relator relies on four categories of allegations in the amended complaint, which he contends state with particularity that Takeda caused false claims to be presented to the government for payment. We address each set of allegations in turn, and conclude that, individually as well as collectively, Relator's allegations fail to allege an essential element of a claim under the Act.

First, Relator alleges in the amended complaint that Takeda promoted Kapidex to rheumatologists, who do not treat the conditions for which Kapidex has been approved. According to Relator, when promoting Kapidex to rheumatologists, Takeda sales representatives equated Kapidex with Prevacid, even though Kapidex was not approved for 10 of the 13 indications for which Prevacid was approved, including the gastric conditions commonly suffered by rheumatology patients. Relator further alleges that Takeda sales representatives were instructed to promote Kapidex to rheumatologists without disclosing that the drug is not approved for the gastric condition often experienced by rheumatology patients.

These allegations concerning the promotion of Kapidex to rheumatologists fall far short of the pleading standards set forth in Rule 9(b) and in Iqbal. Fatal to the claim, Relator does not allege in the amended complaint that the targeted rheumatologists wrote any off-label prescriptions that were submitted to the government for payment, a critical omission in a case brought under the Act. (holding that a complaint does not meet the requirements of Rule 9 when the complaint did not "give notice to the defendant of false claims submitted by others for federal reimbursement of off-label uses, only of illegal practices in promotion of the drug"), overruled on other grounds by Allison Engine Co. v. United ex rel. Sanders. Accordingly, Relator has not plausibly alleged that Takeda caused rheumatologists to write Kapidex prescriptions for off-label uses that actually were presented to the government for payment.

Second, in the amended complaint, Relator identifies 16 primary care physicians (PCPs) who received 60 mg samples of Kapidex from Takeda and collectively wrote 98 prescriptions for the drug that were submitted to the government for reimbursement. Although Relator alleges that these claims were presented to the government for payment, Relator does not plausibly allege that the prescriptions were written for off-label uses.

Rather, Relator alleges in the amended complaint that because PCPs generally do not treat active cases of EE, the only condition for which a 60 mg dose is indicated, any 60 mg prescriptions written by PCPs necessarily were for off-label uses. Notably, however, Relator does not allege facts that specifically address the dosage level of any of the 98 prescriptions. Instead, Relator relies on speculative contentions regarding the 98 prescriptions he has identified. Relator alleges that physicians tend to prescribe drugs in the same dose as the sample the patient has received and that, therefore, the identified PCPs must have prescribed 60 mg doses because they received only 60 mg samples. The allegations in the amended complaint contain the additional speculative assertion that at least 90 percent of the 98 prescriptions must have been written at the 60 mg level, because 93 percent of the overall sales of Kapidex are for dosages of 60 mg.

As the district court observed, Relator fails to state any plausible allegation connecting these general statistics to the 98 prescriptions identified or to prescriptions written by PCPs generally. To the contrary, drawing on the language in the amended complaint, it is logical to assume that a much lower-than-average percentage of the 98 prescriptions were written for 60 mg doses, given that PCPs purportedly do not treat the condition for which the higher 60 mg dose is indicated. Relator also fails to allege directly that any of the identified prescriptions were for off-label uses, instead requiring that a court draw an implausible inference linking general statistics to the 98 prescriptions for Kapidex. (upholding dismissal of False Claims Act claim for lack of particularity because statistical studies cited by the relator did not "directly implicate defendants").

Moreover, even if Relator had pleaded adequately that the 98 prescriptions were written at the 60 mg dosage level, the existence of a 60 mg prescription written by a PCP would not itself constitute a plausible allegation that the prescription was for an off-label use. PCPs can still prescribe a 60 mg dose for an approved use, even though such physicians allegedly do not typically treat the approved condition. This possibility highlights the weakness in the amended complaint, namely, Relator's attempt to draw inferences from general facts, such as that PCPs generally do not treat active cases of EE and that Kapidex generally is prescribed in 60 mg doses, to reach the conclusion that the 98 prescriptions identified in the amended complaint were for off-label uses. We conclude that such inferences are implausible and unsupported by the stated facts and, thus, that the allegations relating to the PCPs do not state with particularity that any false claims were submitted to the government for payment.

Third, Relator alleges in the amended complaint that about 9,000 Kapidex prescriptions were submitted to the government for reimbursement in two of Takeda's sales districts during certain one-year periods. Again, Relator does not allege the dosages of these prescriptions, nor, as the district court observed, do these generalized statistics "identify the types of doctors issuing the prescriptions, the types of illnesses for which they issued the prescriptions at issue, or whether the doctors were subjected to Takeda's sample distribution practices." Thus, the references in the amended complaint to these 9,000 prescriptions do not constitute plausible allegations that Takeda caused presentment of a false claim to the government.

Fourth, in the amended complaint, Relator relies on allegations that are based on the affidavits of two gastroenterologists and one PCP, who averred that they prescribed 60 mg dosages of Kapidex to treat GERD in Medicare patients and were unaware that the drug was available in a 30 mg dosage due to Takeda's sampling practices. However, the amended complaint does not include any details about the particular prescriptions these physicians wrote for Medicare patients, such as approximate dates or patient information, nor does the amended complaint contain allegations that the Medicare patients ever "filled" these prescriptions or that corresponding claims for reimbursement ever were submitted to the government.

As previously discussed, liability under the Act attaches only to false claims actually submitted to the government for reimbursement. General allegations such as those made here, that unidentified Medicare patients received prescriptions for off-label uses, do not identify with particularity any claims that would trigger liability under the Act. In the absence of the required specific allegations, a court is unable to infer that a Medicare patient who has received a prescription for an off-label use actually filled the prescription and sought reimbursement from the government. Indeed, "it may be that physicians prescribed the drug for off-label uses only where the patients paid for it themselves or when the patients' private insurers paid for it." We therefore disagree with Relator's assertion that, if a patient is insured under a government program, we reasonably may infer that any prescription the patient received for an off-label use was filled and that a claim was presented to the government. For these reasons, we conclude that Relator's allegations in the amended complaint relating to the three physician affidavits do not adequately state that any false claims were presented to the government for payment.

Based on our consideration of the facts stated in the amended complaint, we observe that Relator essentially has alleged that some claims must have been presented to the government for payment, because prescriptions of this kind frequently and routinely are obtained by persons who participate in health care programs sponsored by the federal government, or because federally insured patients received off-label prescriptions. As we have explained, allegations of this type are insufficient because they are inherently speculative in nature. In contrast to cases such as Grubbs, Relator's claim does not involve an integrated scheme in which presentment of a claim for payment was a necessary result. We therefore hold that Relator has failed to plead with particularity a plausible claim that any off-label prescriptions were presented to the government for payment.

IV.

Finally, Relator challenges the district court's denial of his motion for leave to amend his complaint for a fourth time. We review the district court's denial of this motion for abuse of discretion. Federal Rule of Civil Procedure 15(a)(2) provides that a court "should freely give leave" to amend a complaint "when justice so requires." Despite this general rule liberally allowing amendments, we have held that a district court may deny leave to amend if the amendment "would be prejudicial to the opposing party, there has been bad faith on the part of the moving party, or the amendment would have been futile."

Relator has amended his complaint three times. A decision granting him leave to amend yet again would have resulted in a fifth complaint filed in this case. We also observe that two years have elapsed between the filing of the original complaint and the district court's dismissal of the amended complaint currently before us in this appeal. The granting of leave to file another amended complaint, when Relator was on notice of the deficiencies before filing the most recent amended complaint, would undermine the substantial interest of finality in litigation and unduly subject Takeda to the continued time and expense occasioned by Relator's pleading failures. In view of the multiple opportunities Relator has been afforded to correct his pleading deficiencies and the deference due to the district court's decision, we conclude that the district court did not abuse its discretion in denying him leave to file a fourth amended complaint.

V.

For these reasons, we hold that the district court properly dismissed the amended complaint under Rule 12(b)(6) for failure to state a claim, and did not abuse its discretion in denying Relator leave to file a fourth amended complaint.

AFFIRMED.

AFFIRMED BY PUBLISHED OPINION. Judge KEENAN wrote the opinion, in which Judge MOTZ and Judge BREDAR joined.

THE FOLLOWING version is the original

UNITED STATES COURT OF APPEALS, FOURTH Circuit.

UNITED STATES ex rel. Noah NATHAN, On Behalf Of The United States Government and the States, Plaintiff–Appellant, v. TAKEDA PHARMACEUTICALS NORTH AMERICA, INCORPORATED; Takeda Pharmaceuticals America, Incorporated, Defendants–Appellees.

No. 11–2077.

Decided: January 11, 2013

Before MOTZ and KEENAN, Circuit Judges, and James K. BREDAR, United States District Judge for the District of Maryland, sitting by designation.ARGUED:Jeffrey A. Lamken, Mololamken, LLP, Washington, D.C., for Appellant. William F. Cavanaugh, Jr., Patterson, Belknap, Webb & Tyler, New York, New York, for Appellees. ON BRIEF:Michael G. Pattillo, Jr., Martin V. Totaro, Mololamken, LLP, Washington, D.C., for Appellant. Susan R. Podolsky, The Law Offices of Susan R. Podolsky, Alexandria, Virginia; Daniel S. Ruzumna, Sean H. Murray, Aileen M. McGill, Patterson, Belknap, Webb & Tyler, New York, New York, for Appellees.

OPINION

Noah Nathan (Relator), a sales manager for Takeda Pharmaceuticals (Takeda), brought this qui tam action against his employer under the False Claims Act (the Act), 31 U.S.C. §§ 3729 through 3733. Relator alleges that Takeda violated § 3729(a)(1)(A) of the Act by causing false claims to be presented to the government for payment under Medicare and other federal health insurance programs.1 After allowing Relator to file a third amended complaint (the amended complaint), the district court dismissed Relator's claims under Federal Rule of Civil Procedure 12(b)(6). In this appeal, Relator argues that the district court erred in concluding that Relator did not plausibly allege in the amended complaint that false claims had been presented to the government for payment, or that Takeda caused the presentment of any such false claims. Relator also contends that the district court abused its discretion in denying Relator's request for leave to file a fourth amended complaint.

Upon our review, we hold that the district court did not err in dismissing the amended complaint, because Relator failed to plausibly allege that any false claims had been presented to the government for payment. We further hold that the district court did not abuse its discretion in denying Relator leave to file a fourth amended complaint.

I.

Among other things, the Act prohibits any person from knowingly "caus[ing] to be presented" to the government false claims for payment or approval. 31 U.S.C. § 3729(a)(1)(A). A false statement is actionable under the Act only if it constitutes a "false or fraudulent claim." Harrison v. Westinghouse Savannah River Co., 176 F.3d 776, 785 (4th Cir.1999) (emphasis added). Importantly, to trigger liability under the Act, a claim actually must have been submitted to the federal government for reimbursement, resulting in "a call upon the government fisc." Id.; see also Hopper v. Solvay Pharm., Inc., 588 F.3d 1318, 1325–26 (11th Cir.2009).

Relator alleges in the amended complaint that prescriptions written for certain medical uses, which have not been approved by the Food and Drug Administration (the FDA) or included in statutorily specified compendia, are not reimbursable under federal health insurance programs. Such uses commonly are referred to as "off-label" uses. Relator further alleges that because the cost of prescriptions for off-label uses is not subject to reimbursement by the federal government, the presentment of these types of claims for payment constitutes a violation of the Act.2

In the amended complaint, Relator additionally alleges that Takeda marketed its prescription drug Kapidex, a proton pump inhibitor used to treat various gastric conditions, for off-label uses.3 Relator alleges that two of Takeda's marketing practices caused presentation of false claims to the government. The identified marketing practices were: (1) Takeda's promotion of Kapidex to rheumatologists, who typically do not treat patients having conditions for which Kapidex has been approved; and (2) Takeda's practice of marketing high doses of Kapidex for the treatment of conditions for which only a lower dose has been approved by the FDA.

In particular, Relator alleges that 60 mg doses of Kapidex have been approved by the FDA only for the treatment of the active condition of erosive esophagitis (EE). However, Kapidex has been approved by the FDA at a lower 30 mg dose to treat the more common condition of gastroesophogeal reflux disease (GERD), as well as for the maintenance of already "healed" cases of EE. Relator alleges that Takeda has provided doctors with samples of Kapidex exclusively in 60 mg doses, irrespective whether such physicians treat active cases of EE. As Relator further alleges, by this sampling practice, Takeda improperly implies that a 60 mg dose of Kapidex is the only available dosage of that drug, thereby causing doctors to prescribe 60 mg doses for unapproved conditions.4 Relator also alleges that Takeda sales representatives regularly misled physicians by deflecting or dismissing their questions about proper dosages, and by making misrepresentations concerning the available dosages.

Additionally, Relator alleges that the motivation for Takeda's alleged fraudulent marketing stems from Takeda's desire to replicate the success of its previously approved drug, Prevacid, the patent for which was set to expire in 2009. Prevacid has been approved to treat 13 conditions, including GERD. Prevacid also has been approved to provide gastric protection and to treat gastric ulcers, indications relevant to rheumatology patients who regularly take anti-inflammatory pain medications. In contrast, Kapidex is not approved for these two conditions. Relator alleges that because the patent expiration date for Prevacid was approaching, Takeda promoted Kapidex to "fill the Prevacid void."

The district court dismissed the amended complaint on two independent grounds: (1) the amended complaint failed to allege the "presentment" of a false or fraudulent claim to the government for payment or approval under 31 U.S.C. § 3729(a)(1)(A); and (2) the amended complaint failed to allege adequately that Takeda "caused" the issuance of off-label prescriptions.5 The district court also denied Relator's request to amend his complaint for a fourth time. Because we conclude that the district court properly dismissed the amended complaint based on Relator's failure to allege presentment of a false claim, we do not reach the additional question whether Relator alleged sufficient facts to support the required causation element for a claim asserted under the Act. We further hold that the district court did not abuse its discretion in denying Relator's motion for leave to file a fourth amended complaint.

II.

We review de novo the district court's dismissal of a complaint for failure to state a claim under Fed.R.Civ.P. 12(b)(6). Harrison, 176 F.3d at 783. To survive a Rule 12(b)(6) motion to dismiss, a complaint must "state a claim to relief that is plausible on its face." Ashcroft v. Iqbal, 556 U.S. 662, 678 (2009) (citation omitted). Facts that are "merely consistent with" liability do not establish a plausible claim to relief. Id . (citation omitted). In addition, although we must view the facts alleged in the light most favorable to the plaintiff, we will not accept "legal conclusions couched as facts or unwarranted inferences, unreasonable conclusions, or arguments." Wag More Dogs, LLC v. Cozart, 680 F.3d 359, 365 (4th Cir.2012) (citation and internal quotation marks omitted).

Before addressing the substantive allegations in the amended complaint, we first state the pleading requirements for fraud-based claims brought under the Act. In addition to meeting the plausibility standard of Iqbal, fraud claims under the Act must be pleaded with particularity pursuant to Rule 9(b) of the Federal Rules of Civil Procedure. Harrison, 176 F.3d at 783–85. Rule 9(b) provides:

In alleging fraud or mistake, a party must state with particularity the circumstances constituting fraud or mistake. Malice, intent, knowledge, and other conditions of a person's mind may be alleged generally.

To satisfy Rule 9(b), a plaintiff asserting a claim under the Act "must, at a minimum, describe the time, place, and contents of the false representations, as well as the identity of the person making the misrepresentation and what he obtained thereby."

United States ex rel. Wilson v. Kellogg Brown & Root, Inc., 525 F.3d 370, 379 (4th Cir.2008) (citation and internal quotation marks omitted).

The parties dispute the proper application of Rule 9(b) in this case. In Relator's view, to meet the requirements for pleading a fraud claim under the Act, a relator need only allege the existence of a fraudulent scheme that supports the inference that false claims were presented to the government for payment. In contrast, Takeda argues that Rule 9(b) requires that a relator plead facts plausibly alleging that particular, identifiable false claims actually were presented to the government for payment.

In view of the rationale underlying Rule 9(b), we decline to adopt Relator's argument for a more lenient application of the Rule. We have adhered firmly to the strictures of Rule 9(b) in applying its terms to cases brought under the Act. See, e.g., Wilson, 525 F.3d at 379–80 (explaining the requirements of Rule 9(b) and affirming dismissal for failing to comply); Harrison, 176 F.3d at 784, 789–90 (same). The multiple purposes of Rule 9(b), namely, of providing notice to a defendant of its alleged misconduct, of preventing frivolous suits, of "eliminat[ing] fraud actions in which all the facts are learned after discovery," and of "protect[ing] defendants from harm to their goodwill and reputation," Harrison, 176 F.3d at 784 (citation omitted), are as applicable in cases brought under the Act as they are in other fraud cases. Indeed, such purposes may apply with particular force in the context of the Act, given the potential consequences flowing from allegations of fraud by companies who transact business with the government. Moreover, we have emphasized that a claim brought under the Act that "rest[s] primarily on facts learned through the costly process of discovery . is precisely what Rule 9(b) seeks to prevent." Wilson, 525 F.3d at 380; see also Harrison, 176 F.3d at 789. For these reasons, nothing in the Act or in our customary application of Rule 9(b) suggests that a more relaxed pleading standard is appropriate in this case.

Neither are we persuaded by Relator's contention that allegations of a fraudulent scheme, in the absence of an assertion that a specific false claim was presented to the government for payment, is a sufficient basis on which to plead a claim under the Act in compliance with Rule 9(b). As the Supreme Court has cautioned, the Act "was not designed to punish every type of fraud committed upon the government." Harrison, 176 F.3d at 785 (citing United States v. McNinch, 356 U.S. 595, 599 (1958)). Instead, the critical question is whether the defendant caused a false claim to be presented to the government, because liability under the Act attaches only to a claim actually presented to the government for payment, not to the underlying fraudulent scheme. Id. (citing United States v. Rivera, 55 F.3d 703, 709 (1st Cir.1995)). Therefore, when a relator fails to plead plausible allegations of presentment, the relator has not alleged all the elements of a claim under the Act. See United States ex rel. Clausen v. Lab. Corp. of Am., 290 F.3d 1301, 1313 (11th Cir.2002) ("[W]e cannot be left wondering whether a plaintiff has offered mere conjecture or a specifically pleaded allegation on an essential element of the lawsuit.").

We agree with the Eleventh Circuit's observation that the particularity requirement of Rule 9(b) "does not permit a False Claims Act plaintiff merely to describe a private scheme in detail but then to allege simply and without any stated reason for his belief that claims requesting illegal payments must have been submitted, were likely submitted or should have been submitted to the Government." Id. at 1311. Rather, Rule 9(b) requires that "some indicia of reliability" must be provided in the complaint to support the allegation that an actual false claim was presented to the government. Id. Indeed, without such plausible allegations of presentment, a relator not only fails to meet the particularity requirement of Rule 9(b), but also does not satisfy the general plausibility standard of Iqbal. See Clausen, 290 F.3d at 1313 ("If Rule 9(b) is to carry any water, it must mean that an essential allegation and circumstance of fraudulent conduct cannot be alleged in such conclusory fashion."); cf. United States ex rel. Joshi v. St. Luke's Hosp., Inc., 441 F.3d 552, 557 (8th Cir.2006) (requiring relator to "provide some representative examples of [the defendants'] alleged fraudulent conduct").

Our conclusion is not altered by the cases cited by Relator, in which courts have held that the requirements of Rule 9(b) can be satisfied in the absence of particularized allegations of specific false claims. Based on the nature of the schemes alleged in many of those cases, specific allegations of the defendant's fraudulent conduct necessarily led to the plausible inference that false claims were presented to the government.

For example, in United States ex rel. Grubbs v. Kanneganti, 565 F.3d 180 (5th Cir.2009), the relator alleged a conspiracy by doctors to seek reimbursement from governmental health programs for services that never were performed. The court concluded that, because the complaint included the dates of specific services that were recorded by the physicians but never were provided, such allegations constituted "more than probable, nigh likely, circumstantial evidence that the doctors' fraudulent records caused the hospital's billing system in due course to present fraudulent claims to the Government." Id. at 192. Accordingly, the court further concluded that it would "stretch the imagination" for the doctors to continually record services that were not provided, but "to deviate from the regular billing track at the last moment so that the recorded, but unprovided, services never get billed." Id.; see also United States ex rel. Duxbury v. Ortho Biotech Prods., L.P., 579 F.3d 13, 30 (1st Cir.2009) (holding that, in scheme alleging kickbacks to health care providers, allegations regarding "the dates and amounts of the false claims filed by these providers with the Medicare program" met the standard imposed by Rule 9(b)).6

Applying these principles, we hold that when a defendant's actions, as alleged and as reasonably inferred from the allegations, could have led, but need not necessarily have led, to the submission of false claims, a relator must allege with particularity that specific false claims actually were presented to the government for payment. To the extent that other cases apply a more relaxed construction of Rule 9(b) in such circumstances, we disagree with that approach.

In reaching this conclusion, we acknowledge the practical challenges that a relator may face in cases such as the present one, in which a relator may not have independent access to records such as prescription invoices, and where privacy laws may pose a barrier to obtaining such information without court involvement. Nevertheless, our pleading requirements do not permit a relator to bring an action without pleading facts that support all the elements of a claim. See Dickson v. Microsoft Corp., 309 F.3d 193, 213 (4th Cir.2002) (noting "the basic pleading requirement that a plaintiff set forth facts sufficient to allege each element of his claim"). We further emphasize, however, that the standard we articulate today does not foreclose claims under the Act when a relator plausibly pleads that specific, identifiable claims actually were presented to the government for payment. Of course, whether such factual allegations in a given case meet the required standard must be evaluated on a case-specific basis.

III.

Employing the above pleading standard, we turn to consider the sufficiency of the amended complaint in this case. Relator relies on four categories of allegations in the amended complaint, which he contends state with particularity that Takeda caused false claims to be presented to the government for payment. We address each set of allegations in turn, and conclude that, individually as well as collectively, Relator's allegations fail to allege an essential element of a claim under the Act.

First, Relator alleges in the amended complaint that Takeda promoted Kapidex to rheumatologists, who do not treat the conditions for which Kapidex has been approved.7 According to Relator, when promoting Kapidex to rheumatologists, Takeda sales representatives equated Kapidex with Prevacid, even though Kapidex was not approved for 10 of the 13 indications for which Prevacid was approved, including the gastric conditions commonly suffered by rheumatology patients. Relator further alleges that Takeda sales representatives were instructed to promote Kapidex to rheumatologists without disclosing that the drug is not approved for the gastric condition often experienced by rheumatology patients.

These allegations concerning the promotion of Kapidex to rheumatologists fall far short of the pleading standards set forth in Rule 9(b) and in Iqbal. Fatal to the claim, Relator does not allege in the amended complaint that the targeted rheumatologists wrote any off-label prescriptions that were submitted to the government for payment, a critical omission in a case brought under the Act.8 See United States ex rel. Rost v. Pfizer, Inc., 507 F.3d 720, 733 (1st Cir.2007) (holding that a complaint does not meet the requirements of Rule 9 when the complaint did not "give notice to [the defendant] of false claims submitted by others for federal reimbursement of off-label uses, only of illegal practices in promotion of the drug"), overruled on other grounds by Allison Engine Co. v. United ex rel. Sanders, 553 U.S. 662 (2008). Accordingly, Relator has not plausibly alleged that Takeda caused rheumatologists to write Kapidex prescriptions for off-label uses that actually were presented to the government for payment.

Second, in the amended complaint, Relator identifies 16 primary care physicians (PCPs) who received 60 mg samples of Kapidex from Takeda and collectively wrote 98 prescriptions for the drug that were submitted to the government for reimbursement. Although Relator alleges that these claims were presented to the government for payment, Relator does not plausibly allege that the prescriptions were written for off-label uses.

Rather, Relator alleges in the amended complaint that because PCPs generally do not treat active cases of EE, the only condition for which a 60 mg dose is indicated, any 60 mg prescriptions written by PCPs necessarily were for off-label uses. Notably, however, Relator does not allege facts that specifically address the dosage level of any of the 98 prescriptions. Instead, Relator relies on speculative contentions regarding the 98 prescriptions he has identified. Relator alleges that physicians tend to prescribe drugs in the same dose as the sample the patient has received and that, therefore, the identified PCPs must have prescribed 60 mg doses because they received only 60 mg samples. The allegations in the amended complaint contain the additional speculative assertion that at least 90 percent of the 98 prescriptions must have been written at the 60 mg level, because 93 percent of the overall sales of Kapidex are for dosages of 60 mg.

As the district court observed, Relator fails to state any plausible allegation connecting these general statistics to the 98 prescriptions identified or to prescriptions written by PCPs generally. To the contrary, drawing on the language in the amended complaint, it is logical to assume that a much lower-than-average percentage of the 98 prescriptions were written for 60 mg doses, given that PCPs purportedly do not treat the condition for which the higher 60 mg dose is indicated. Relator also fails to allege directly that any of the identified prescriptions were for off-label uses, instead requiring that a court draw an implausible inference linking general statistics to the 98 prescriptions for Kapidex. Cf. United States ex rel. Thompson v. Columbia/HCA Healthcare Corp., 125 F.3d 899, 903 (5th Cir.1997) (upholding dismissal of False Claims Act claim for lack of particularity because statistical studies cited by the relator did not "directly implicate defendants").

Moreover, even if Relator had pleaded adequately that the 98 prescriptions were written at the 60 mg dosage level, the existence of a 60 mg prescription written by a PCP would not itself constitute a plausible allegation that the prescription was for an off-label use. PCPs can still prescribe a 60 mg dose for an approved use, even though such physicians allegedly do not typically treat the approved condition. This possibility highlights the weakness in the amended complaint, namely, Relator's attempt to draw inferences from general facts, such as that PCPs generally do not treat active cases of EE and that Kapidex generally is prescribed in 60 mg doses, to reach the conclusion that the 98 prescriptions identified in the amended complaint were for off-label uses. We conclude that such inferences are implausible and unsupported by the stated facts and, thus, that the allegations relating to the PCPs do not state with particularity that any false claims were submitted to the government for payment.

Third, Relator alleges in the amended complaint that about 9,000 Kapidex prescriptions were submitted to the government for reimbursement in two of Takeda's sales districts during certain one-year periods. Again, Relator does not allege the dosages of these prescriptions, nor, as the district court observed, do these generalized statistics "identify the types of doctors issuing the prescriptions, the types of illnesses for which they issued the prescriptions at issue, or whether the doctors were subjected to Takeda's sample distribution practices." Thus, the references in the amended complaint to these 9,000 prescriptions do not constitute plausible allegations that Takeda caused presentment of a false claim to the government.

Fourth, in the amended complaint, Relator relies on allegations that are based on the affidavits of two gastroenterologists and one PCP, who averred that they prescribed 60 mg dosages of Kapidex to treat GERD in Medicare patients and were unaware that the drug was available in a 30 mg dosage due to Takeda's sampling practices. However, the amended complaint does not include any details about the particular prescriptions these physicians wrote for Medicare patients, such as approximate dates or patient information, nor does the amended complaint contain allegations that the Medicare patients ever "filled" these prescriptions or that corresponding claims for reimbursement ever were submitted to the government.9

As previously discussed, liability under the Act attaches only to false claims actually submitted to the government for reimbursement. General allegations such as those made here, that unidentified Medicare patients received prescriptions for off-label uses, do not identify with particularity any claims that would trigger liability under the Act. In the absence of the required specific allegations, a court is unable to infer that a Medicare patient who has received a prescription for an off-label use actually filled the prescription and sought reimbursement from the government. Indeed, "[i]t may be that physicians prescribed [the drug] for off-label uses only where the patients paid for it themselves or when the patients' private insurers paid for it." Rost, 507 F.3d at 733. We therefore disagree with Relator's assertion that, if a patient is insured under a government program, we reasonably may infer that any prescription the patient received for an off-label use was filled and that a claim was presented to the government. For these reasons, we conclude that Relator's allegations in the amended complaint relating to the three physician affidavits do not adequately state that any false claims were presented to the government for payment.

Based on our consideration of the facts stated in the amended complaint, we observe that Relator essentially has alleged that some claims must have been presented to the government for payment, because prescriptions of this kind frequently and routinely are obtained by persons who participate in health care programs sponsored by the federal government, or because federally insured patients received off-label prescriptions. As we have explained, allegations of this type are insufficient because they are inherently speculative in nature. In contrast to cases such as Grubbs, 565 F.3d 180, Relator's claim does not involve an integrated scheme in which presentment of a claim for payment was a necessary result. We therefore hold that Relator has failed to plead with particularity a plausible claim that any off-label prescriptions were presented to the government for payment.

IV.

Finally, Relator challenges the district court's denial of his motion for leave to amend his complaint for a fourth time. We review the district court's denial of this motion for abuse of discretion. Wilson, 525 F.3d at 376. Federal Rule of Civil Procedure 15(a)(2) provides that a court "should freely give leave" to amend a complaint "when justice so requires." Despite this general rule liberally allowing amendments, we have held that a district court may deny leave to amend if the amendment "would be prejudicial to the opposing party, there has been bad faith on the part of the moving party, or the amendment would have been futile." Laber v. Harvey, 438 F.3d 404, 426 (4th Cir.2006) (en banc) (quoting Johnson v. Oroweat Foods Co., 785 F.2d 503, 509 (4th Cir.1986)).

Relator has amended his complaint three times. A decision granting him leave to amend yet again would have resulted in a fifth complaint filed in this case. We also observe that two years have elapsed between the filing of the original complaint and the district court's dismissal of the amended complaint currently before us in this appeal. The granting of leave to file another amended complaint, when Relator was on notice of the deficiencies before filing the most recent amended complaint,10 would undermine the substantial interest of finality in litigation and unduly subject Takeda to the continued time and expense occasioned by Relator's pleading failures. In view of the multiple opportunities Relator has been afforded to correct his pleading deficiencies and the deference due to the district court's decision, we conclude that the district court did not abuse its discretion in denying him leave to file a fourth amended complaint.

V.

For these reasons, we hold that the district court properly dismissed the amended complaint under Rule 12(b)(6) for failure to state a claim, and did not abuse its discretion in denying Relator leave to file a fourth amended complaint.

AFFIRMED.

FOOTNOTES

1. Relator does not appeal the district court's dismissal of Relator's separate claim brought under 31 U.S.C. § 3729(a)(1)(B).

2. Nevertheless, physicians are permitted to prescribe drugs for off-label uses. See 21 U.S.C. § 396. However, under the Federal Food, Drug, and Cosmetic Act, 21 U.S.C. § 301, et seq., pharmaceutical companies are not permitted to promote their drugs for uses not approved by the FDA. See Wash. Legal Found. v. Henney, 202 F.3d 331, 332–33 (D.C.Cir.2000).

3. Relator alleges that Kapidex has been renamed Dexilant. Because the amended complaint refers to the drug at issue exclusively as Kapidex, we do the same here.

4. Relator alleges that although Takeda sought government approval for higher dosages of Kapidex, including a 60 mg dose to treat GERD, the Food and Drug Administration rejected this request.

5. Because Relator does not appeal the district court's decision declining to exercise supplemental jurisdiction over Relator's state law claims, we do not address those claims here.

6. In another case cited by Relator, the Tenth Circuit held that "claims under the [False Claims Act] need only show the specifics of a fraudulent scheme and provide an adequate basis for a reasonable inference that false claims were submitted as part of that scheme." United States ex rel. Lemmon v. Envirocare of Utah, Inc., 614 F.3d 1163, 1172 (10th Cir.2010). In Lemmon, however, it was clear that the relator had pleaded specific details of false claims, including the dates of the alleged violations, the dates payment requests were submitted, details of the purported violations, and the allegedly false certification language.

7. According to Relator, rheumatologists do not treat GERD or EE, the two indications for which Kapidex is approved.

Rheumatology patients may use Prevacid for gastric protection, a need associated with long-term ingestion of anti-inflammatory drugs such as Advil. However, as discussed above, Kapidex is not approved for gastric protection.

8. After filing the amended complaint, Relator submitted to the district court a supplemental affidavit with attachments, which allegedly showed that two rheumatologists in Relator's sales territory wrote Kapidex prescriptions during a particular month. However, Relator cannot cure pleading deficiencies in the amended complaint with later-filed supporting documentation. See E.I. du Pont de Nemours & Co. v. Kolon Indus., 637 F.3d 435, 448–49 (4th Cir.2011) (explaining that "matters beyond the pleadings . cannot be considered on a Rule 12(b)(6) motion"); Sec'y of State for Defence v. Trimble Navigation Ltd., 484 F.3d 700, 705 (4th Cir .2007) (stating the documents that may be considered in evaluating a Rule 12(b)(6) motion). Moreover, we agree with the district court's observation that, even if these allegations had been included in the amended complaint, "there is nothing that prevents a rheumatologist from prescribing Kapidex for an approved condition at an approved dosage," and there was no indication in the record of the prescriptions' dosage, the conditions for which they were written, or that the prescriptions were submitted to the government for reimbursement.

9. In a supplemental affidavit, Dr. Michael Yaffe, the PCP, averred that he had personal knowledge that some of his Medicare patients filled the off-label Kapidex prescriptions because the patients contacted his office to seek prescription refills. Once again, it is improper for Relator to attempt to buttress his faulty complaint with supplemental affidavits submitted later in the litigation, in this case, in opposition to Takeda's motion to dismiss.

10. In May 2011, the district court dismissed Relator's second amended complaint for failure to state a claim, but granted leave to amend. In its order, the district court noted the lack of specific

allegations regarding actual presentation of false claims to the government. Although the amended complaint before us includes considerably more detail, this fundamental defect was not addressed adequately by the last amendment. The district court also cautioned Relator that any evidence provided outside the amended complaint could not be considered in an attempt to avoid dismissal under Rule 12(b)(6).

AFFIRMED BY PUBLISHED OPINION. Judge KEENAN wrote the opinion, in which Judge MOTZ and Judge BREDAR joined.

18

THE UNITED STATES SUPREME COURT

My petition for a Writ of Certiorari is 44 pages, which makes it hard to put the entire document in this book (the entire document is available online), but I will hit the highlights. In layman's terms, this is the document submitted to ask the U.S. Supreme Court to hear my appeal.

The U.S. Supreme Court will hear about 70 cases per year and decide about another 50 without hearing arguments. They will receive about 7,000 cases per year asking for their review. To accept review, four of the nine justices must vote in favor of a case, I do not know what my vote was?

The Solicitor General is the federal government's lawyer in the Supreme Court. Having the justices send a case to the SG is the least likely scenario for a cert petition, around 20 cases per year. I can at least take some pride that it made it that far.

In the next chapter, I will get into more information about the Solicitor General, including the SG's brief to the Court in my case.

.   .   .

From my Supreme Court Cert Petition (Edited to make it easier to read. The unedited version is at the end of the chapter.)

QUESTION PRESENTED

The False Claims Act provides for the imposition of civil penalties and treble damages against "any person" who "knowingly presents, or causes to be presented, a false or fraudulent claim for payment or approval" by the United States Government. In "alleging fraud," a complaint "must state with particularity the circumstances constituting fraud." The question presented is:

Whether Rule 9(b) requires that a complaint under the False Claims Act "allege with particularity that specific false claims actually were presented to the government for payment," as required by the Fourth, Sixth, Eighth, and Eleventh Circuits, or whether it is instead sufficient to allege the "particular details of" the "scheme to submit false claims" together with sufficient indicia that false claims were submitted, as held by the First, Fifth, Seventh, and Ninth Circuits.

B. Prescription Reimbursement Under Federal Health Benefits Programs

The federal government annually pays billions of dollars for healthcare services through Medicare and Medicaid. Medicare is "a federally funded medical insurance program for the elderly and disabled," while Medicaid "authorizes federal financial assistance to States" to help cover "costs of medical treatment for needy persons."

A prescription's eligibility for reimbursement under those federal programs turns primarily on the scope of the FDA's approval. We therefore briefly describe the regulatory scheme under the Food, Drug, and Cosmetic Act ("FDCA"), before turning to reimbursement criteria under federal healthcare programs.

2. Eligibility For Reimbursement

UNDER MEDICAID AND MEDICARE, a prescription is reimbursable only if used for a "medically accepted indication." If the FDA has approved the medication for the patient's condition, the use is a "medically accepted indication." An "off-label" use—a use the FDA has not approved—may qualify as a "medically accepted indication," but only under one condition: The use must be supported by one of the drug compendia specified in the relevant statutes.

Thus, if a drug is prescribed for an FDA-approved use, or for an "off-label" use supported by one of the drug compendia, it is for a "medically accepted indication" and reimbursable under Medicaid and Medicare. By contrast, drugs prescribed for uses neither approved by the FDA nor supported by the compendia are not for medically accepted indications and are not reimbursable.

B. This Case Presents An Appropriate Vehicle For Resolving The Conflict

This case presents an excellent vehicle for resolving the circuit conflict. The case exhibits none of the jurisdictional impediments that weighed against review in Duxbury. Moreover, the choice of pleading standard was outcome-determinative. The Fourth Circuit affirmed the dismissal on the grounds that the Complaint does not "allege with particularity that specific false claims actually were presented to the government for payment." And it so held even though the Complaint "alleges particular details of a scheme to submit false claims paired with reliable indicia that lead to a strong inference that claims actually were submitted," that are sufficient under the standard applied by the First, Fifth, Seventh, and Ninth Circuits.

The gravamen of the Complaint is that Takeda, by aggressively marketing 60-mg Kapidex for uses that are not medically indicated, "knowingly caused to be presented" numerous "false or fraudulent claims for government payment or approval" in violation of the False Claims Act. The court of appeals did not suggest—nor did Takeda argue—that the Complaint failed to "allege particular details" of Takeda's "scheme to submit false claims." The Complaint contains extensive allegations, including references to Takeda internal documents and doctor affidavits, detailing Takeda's promotion of Kapidex at double the medically indicated dosage for GERD to physicians who ordinarily would not treat anything but GERD. Indeed, Takeda provided samples at only 60 mg even though GERD—the dominant use by a 10-to-1 ratio—was approved only at a 30-mg dose. And the court of appeals never suggested, and Takeda has never argued, that 60-mg Kapidex prescriptions for GERD would not constitute false claims within the meaning of the False Claims Act when submitted for reimbursement.

Because the relator is not a doctor prescribing Kapidex, a patient taking Kapidex, or a pharmacist filling Kapidex prescriptions—and because privacy laws prevent third parties from accessing such records, he was unable to produce the individual off- label prescriptions or requests for reimbursement themselves. Under the First, Fifth, Seventh, and Ninth Circuits' standard, the Complaint would be sufficient so long as it contains "reliable indicia that lead to a strong inference that claims actually were submitted." It plainly does. Among other things, the Complaint incorporates affidavits from three doctors confirming relator's theory of the case. Each of those doctors—including board-certified gastroenterologists, one of whom is a former President of the American Medical Association—attests that, because of Takeda's aggressive marketing of 60-mg Kapidex and sampling exclusively at that dose, they were unaware that Kapidex came in a 30-mg dose. And they expressly state that Takeda's 60-mg sampling influenced them to write Kapidex prescriptions for GERD at 60 mg, even though that is not a medically accepted indication.

The Fourth Circuit rejected that evidence because the Complaint did "not include any details about the particular prescriptions these physicians wrote for Medicare patients, such as approximate dates or patient information." But Nathan used the means available to him to identify 98 specific prescriptions, written by 16 named primary-care physicians, that the Complaint alleges are "specific examples of certain false claims." For each prescription, the Complaint identifies the treating physician; provides the dates the physician received 60-mg Kapidex samples from Takeda; specifies the month the prescription was written; and alleges that it was submitted to Medicare for reimbursement. For example, the Complaint alleges that "Dr. (Z*) wrote 2 prescriptions * * * , including 1 prescription for Kapidex in August 2010 and 1 in September 2010"; that they were "submitted to Medicare for reimbursement during the identified 6-month period"; and that "Dr. (Z*) received Kapidex 60 mg samples on * * * August 26, 2010, and November 4, 2010." The Complaint does likewise for 15 other physicians and 96 other prescriptions.

Because the Complaint alleges that primary-care physicians treat GERD but not EE, the most reasonable inference is that the 98 prescriptions were written for GERD. And because, as the Complaint makes clear, 93% of all Kapidex prescriptions are written at 60 mg, and because physicians prescribe PPIs in the dose being sampled, "one may deduce" that there is a "more than 90%" certainty that each of those 98 GERD prescriptions was "written at the 60 mg dose," a dosage for which it is not medically indicated and hence not reimbursable. Thus, even without providing all of the "details as to each false claim," the Complaint provides ample "factual and statistical evidence" that "strengthens the inference of fraud beyond mere possibility." That is sufficient to satisfy Rule 9(b) as applied by the First, Fifth, Seventh, and Ninth Circuits.

By contrast, in the absence of specific allegations that the 98 prescriptions actually were written for GERD at 60 mg and thus were non-reimbursable, in other words, allegations sufficient to prove the False Claims Act violation—the Fourth Circuit refused "to draw inferences from general facts." To the contrary, the court consistently assumed the opposite of what the "general facts" would show, speculating that the 98 prescriptions might be such outliers that not even one was written for GERD at 60 mg, and hence a false claim when submitted to Medicare. For example, the court of appeals refused to credit the allegation that it was 93% likely that those prescriptions were for 60-mg doses because, in its view, the overall 93% rate of 60-mg versus 30-mg prescriptions might not apply to those particular prescriptions. And the court simply ignored the Complaint's allegation regarding the effect of PPI trials—that the prescriptions necessarily would have been written at 60 mg because that is the only dose the doctors had available to conduct PPI trials from physician affidavits incorporated into complaint. But the requirement of particularity is not a license to speculate around and ignore the Complaint's specific allegations.

The court of appeals also speculated that, even though the Complaint specifically alleges that primary-care physicians treat GERD, but do not generally treat EE, it is not plausible that the specifically identified primary-care physicians were writing Kapidex prescriptions for GERD rather than EE. The court noted that it is possible for primary-care physicians to "prescribe a 60 mg dose for an approved use," i.e., for healing EE, and speculated that it was more likely that each of the 98 prescriptions was written for a proper indication. But the Complaint makes the contrary inference—that primary-care physicians were prescribing Kapidex for something they ordinarily treat, and not for something that can be diagnosed only through an endoscopy they would not perform—far more probable. Only under the 9(b)-on-steroids standard the Fourth Circuit adopted could it be said that the Complaint's allegations about the 98 prescriptions "do not state with particularity that any false claims were submitted to the government for payment." The Court should grant review and resolve the well-established conflict on the standard applicable to these sorts of cases.

CONCLUSION

The petition for a writ of certiorari should be granted. Respectfully submitted.

May 2013

JEFFREY A. LAMKEN

Counsel of Record

MICHAEL G. PATTILLO, JR. MOLOLAMKEN LLP

The Watergate, Suite 660 600 New Hampshire Ave.,NW Washington, D.C. 20037 (202) 556-2000 jlamken@molo-lamken.com

Counsel for Petitioner

As I STATED EARLIER, soon after our filing of the case Takeda changed the data provided to the representatives, which clearly shows my physicians were prescribing Dexilant at the 60mg dose but it was too late to enter that information into the case.

FROM MY SUPREME COURT Cert Petition (Original version)

QUESTION PRESENTED

The False Claims Act provides for the imposition of civil penalties and treble damages against "any person" who "knowingly presents, or causes to be presented, a false or fraudulent claim for payment or approval" by the United States Government. 31 U.S.C. § 3729(a)(1)(A). In "alleging fraud," a complaint "must state with particularity the circumstances constituting fraud." Fed. R. Civ. P. 9(b). The question presented is:

Whether Rule 9(b) requires that a complaint under the False Claims Act "allege with particularity that specific false claims actually were presented to the government for payment," as required by the Fourth, Sixth, Eighth, and Eleventh Circuits, or whether it is instead sufficient to allege the "particular details of" the "scheme to submit false claims" together with sufficient indicia that false claims were submitted, as held by the First, Fifth, Seventh, and Ninth Circuits.

B. Prescription Reimbursement Under Federal Health Benefits Programs

The federal government annually pays billions of dollars for healthcare services through Medicare and Medicaid. See Cong. Budget Office, The Long-Term Budget Outlook 21 (2009). Medicare is "a federally funded medical insurance program for the elderly and disabled," Fischer v. United States, 529 U.S. 667, 671 (2000), while Medicaid "authorizes federal financial assistance to States" to help cover "costs of medical treatment for needy persons," Pharm. Research & Mfrs. of Am. v. Walsh, 538 U.S. 644, 650 (2003).

A prescription's eligibility for reimbursement under those federal programs turns primarily on the scope of the FDA's approval. We therefore briefly describe the regulatory scheme under the Food, Drug, and Cosmetic Act ("FDCA"), 21 U.S.C. §§ 301 et seq., before turning to reimbursement criteria under federal healthcare programs.

2. Eligibility For Reimbursement

· · ·

UNDER MEDICAID AND MEDICARE, a prescription is reimbursable only if used for a "medically accepted indication." See 42 U.S.C. §§ 1395w-102(e)(1)(A), 1396b(i)(10), 1396r-8(k)(2)-(3).1 If the FDA has approved the medication for the patient's condition, the use is a "medically accepted indication." Id. § 1396r-8(k)(6). An "off-label" use—a use the FDA has not approved—may qualify as a "medically accepted indication," but only under one condition: The use must be supported by one of the drug compendia specified in the relevant statutes. Ibid. (Medicaid); id. § 1395w-102(e)(4) (Medicare); id. § 1396r- 8(g)(1)(B)(i) (listing compendia).

Thus, if a drug is prescribed for an FDA-approved use, or for an "off-label" use supported by one of the drug compendia, it is for a "medically accepted indication" and reimbursable under Medicaid and Medicare. By contrast, drugs prescribed for uses neither approved by the FDA nor supported by the compendia are not for medically accepted indications and are not reimbursable.

B. THIS CASE Presents An Appropriate Vehicle For Resolving The Conflict

This case presents an excellent vehicle for resolving the circuit conflict. The case exhibits none of the jurisdictional impediments that weighed against review in Duxbury. Moreover, the choice of pleading standard was outcome-determinative. The Fourth Circuit affirmed the dismissal on the grounds that the Complaint does not "allege with particularity that specific false claims actually were presented to the government for payment." App., infra, 10a. And it so held even though the Complaint "alleg[es] particular details of a scheme to submit false claims paired with reliable indicia that lead to a strong inference that claims actually were submitted," Grubbs, 565 F.3d at 190, that are sufficient under the standard applied by the First, Fifth, Seventh, and Ninth Circuits.

The gravamen of the Complaint is that Takeda, by aggressively marketing 60-mg Kapidex for uses that are not medically indicated, "knowingly * * * cause[d] to be presented" numerous "false or fraudulent claim[s] for [government] payment or approval" in violation of the False Claims Act, 31 U.S.C. § 3729(a)(1)(A). The court of appeals did not suggest—nor did Takeda argue—that the Complaint failed to "alleg[e] particular details" of Takeda's "scheme to submit false claims." Grubbs, 565 F.3d at 190. The Complaint contains extensive allegations, including references to Takeda internal documents and doctor affidavits, detailing Takeda's promotion of Kapidex at double the medically indicated dosage for GERD to physicians who ordinarily would not treat anything but GERD. See pp. 7-10, supra. Indeed, Takeda provided samples at only 60 mg even though GERD—the dominant use by a 10-to-1 ratio—was approved only at a 30-mg dose. And the court of appeals never suggested, and Takeda has never argued, that 60-mg Kapidex prescriptions for GERD would not constitute false claims within the meaning of the False Claims Act when submitted for reimbursement.

Because the relator is not a doctor prescribing Kapidex, a patient taking Kapidex, or a pharmacist filling Kapidex prescriptions—and because privacy laws prevent third parties from accessing such records, see App., infra, 10a—he was unable to produce the individual off- label prescriptions or requests for reimbursement themselves. Under the First, Fifth, Seventh, and Ninth Circuits' standard, the Complaint would be sufficient so long as it contains "reliable indicia that lead to a strong inference that claims actually were submitted." Grubbs, 565 F.3d at 190. It plainly does. Among other things, the Complaint incorporates affidavits from three doctors confirming relator's theory of the case. App., infra, 98a- 103a(¶¶273,275,278,279,281);169a-178a. Each of those doctors—including board-certified gastroenterologists, one of whom is a former President of the American Medical Association—attests that, because of Takeda's aggressive marketing of 60-mg Kapidex and sampling exclusively at that dose, they were unaware that Kapidex came in a 30-mg dose. Id. at 44a(¶10); 98a-103a(¶¶273- 281). And they expressly state that Takeda's 60-mg sampling influenced them to write Kapidex prescriptions for GERD at 60 mg, even though that is not a medically accepted indication. Ibid.

The Fourth Circuit rejected that evidence because the Complaint did "not include any details about the particular prescriptions these physicians wrote for Medicare patients, such as approximate dates or patient information." App., infra, 15a. But Nathan used the means available to him to identify 98 specific prescriptions, written by 16 named primary-care physicians, that the Complaint alleges are "specific examples of certain false claims." Id. at 123a (¶ 379). For each prescription, the Complaint identifies the treating physician; provides the dates the physician received 60-mg Kapidex samples from Takeda; specifies the month the prescription was written; and alleges that it was submitted to Medicare for reimbursement. Id. at 105a-109a (¶¶ 286-301). For example, the Complaint alleges that "Dr. (Z*) wrote 2 prescriptions * * * , including 1 prescription for Kapidex in August 2010 and 1 in September 2010"; that they were "submitted to Medicare for reimbursement during [the identified] 6-month period"; and that "Dr. (Z*) received Kapidex 60 mg samples on * * * August 26, 2010, and November 4, 2010." Id. at 107a (¶ 295). The Complaint does likewise for 15 other physicians and 96 other prescriptions. Id.at105a-109a(¶¶286-294,296-301).

Because the Complaint alleges that primary-care physicians treat GERD but not EE, the most reasonable inference is that the 98 prescriptions were written for GERD. App., infra, 84a-85a (¶¶ 206-209). And because, as the Complaint makes clear, 93% of all Kapidex prescriptions are written at 60 mg, id. at 88a(¶228), and because physicians prescribe PPIs in the dose being sampled, id.

at 99a-102a(¶¶278, 281), "one may deduce" that there is a "more than 90%" certainty that each of those 98 GERD prescriptions was "written at the 60 mg dose," id. at 110a(¶310)—a dosage for which it is not medically indicated and hence not reimbursable. Id. at 66a(¶120). Thus, even without providing all of the "details as to each false claim," the Complaint provides ample "factual [and] statistical evidence" that "strengthen[s] the inference of fraud beyond [mere] possibility." Duxbury, 579 F.3d at 29. That is sufficient to satisfy Rule 9(b) as applied by the First, Fifth, Seventh, and Ninth Circuits.

By contrast, in the absence of specific allegations that the 98 prescriptions actually were written for GERD at 60 mg and thus were non-reimbursable—in other words, allegations sufficient to prove the False Claims Act violation—the Fourth Circuit refused "to draw inferences from general facts." App., infra, 14a. To the contrary, the court consistently assumed the opposite of what the "general facts" would show, speculating that the 98 prescriptions might be such outliers that not even one was written for GERD at 60 mg, and hence a false claim when submitted to Medicare. For example, the court of appeals refused to credit the allegation that it was 93% likely that those prescriptions were for 60-mg doses because, in its view, the overall 93% rate of 60-mg versus 30-mg prescriptions might not apply to those particular prescriptions. Id. at 13a-14a. And the court simply ignored the Complaint's allegation regarding the effect of PPI trials—that the prescriptions necessarily would have been written at 60 mg because that is the only dose the doctors had available to conduct PPI trials. Id. at 99a- 102a(¶¶278, 279, 281); id. at 167a, 169a, 173a, 177a (physician affidavits incorporated into complaint). But the requirement of particularity is not a license to speculate around and ignore the Complaint's specific allegations.

The court of appeals also speculated that, even though the Complaint specifically alleges that primary-care physicians treat GERD, but do not generally treat EE, it is not plausible that the specifically identified primary-care physicians were writing Kapidex prescriptions for GERD rather than EE. App., infra, 14a. The court noted that it is possible for primary-care physicians to "prescribe a 60 mg dose for an approved use," i.e., for healing EE, and speculated that it was more likely that each of the 98 prescriptions was written for a proper indication. Ibid. But the Complaint makes the contrary inference—that primary-care physicians were prescribing Kapidex for something they ordinarily treat, and not for something that can be diagnosed only through an endoscopy they would not perform—far more probable. Only under the 9(b)-on-steroids standard the Fourth Circuit adopted could it be said that the Complaint's allegations about the 98 prescriptions "do not state with particularity that any false claims were submitted to the government for payment." Id. at 15a. The Court should grant review and resolve the well-established conflict on the standard applicable to these sorts of cases.

CONCLUSION

The petition for a writ of certiorari should be granted. Respectfully submitted.

May 2013

JEFFREY A. LAMKEN

Counsel of Record

MICHAEL G. PATTILLO, JR. MOLOLAMKEN LLP

The Watergate, Suite 660 600 New Hampshire Ave.,NW Washington, D.C. 20037 (202) 556-2000 jlamken@mololamken.com

Counsel for Petitioner

19

THE SOLICITOR GENERAL OF THE UNITED STATES

The Solicitor General of the United States is the federal government's lawyer in the Supreme Court. In an article by Stephen Wermiel on scotusblog.com[1], he explains that the SG's job requires them to, "strike a sometimes delicate balance between serving the legal interests of his superiors (the President and Attorney General), the long-term interests of the United States (as opposed to the present Administration), and his responsibility as a special officer of the Court itself."

The Solicitor General position was created by Congress in 1870 to consolidate government litigation into one office. Over the years the office has grown to about twenty attorneys. The SG is appointed by the President and confirmed by the Senate. Wermiel[2] points out that the SG is the only position in the "entire federal bureaucracy, including the job of Supreme Court Justice, for which there is a statutory requirement that the appointee must be "learned in the law.""

Of the twenty attorneys in the SG's office, many have gone on to become Supreme Court Justices themselves. Just looking at the current nine justices, Chief Justice John Roberts and Justice

Samuel Alito worked in the office while Justice Elena Kagan was the SG herself.[3]

One way to view the SG's office is as the gatekeeper for the Court. As what happened in my case, the Court will sometimes ask the SG's opinion about an issue of federal law in which the government is not a party. On average, the U.S. Supreme Court will request the SG's opinion about 20 times a year, out of about 7,000 annual cases. Since the government did not intervene in my case as a False Claims Act, I moved forward as a qui tam case on my own but on behalf of the government. As the gatekeeper, the Supreme Court holds the SG's determination in high regards.

Donald B. Verrilli Jr. was the Solicitor General of the United States and the Counsel of Record for the "Brief for the United States *Amicus Curiae*" written in my case. The Brief states, "This brief is submitted in response to the order of the Court inviting the Solicitor General to express the views of the United States. In the view of the United States, the petition for a writ of certiorari should be denied."

It is my opinion that they were concerned with the makeup of the Supreme Court and concerned that if they took my case and ruled against me that the whole country would be bad for whistleblowers. At the time of this brief, there was a circuit court split with half of the United States applying a flexible standard and a half using a strict standard regarding the specificity required under rule 9(b) in False Claims Act whistleblower cases. I feel the flexible standard is what President Abraham Lincoln's intention was when he signed the False Claims Act into law to prevent fraud against the government of the United States.

I will show in the next chapter, *Thomas Foglia v. Renal Ventures Management,* how the Federal 3rd Circuit used the Solicitor General's Brief from my case to reach a favorable decision on the Rule 9(b) issue compared to what the Federal 4th Circuit concluded in my case.

From the *Thomas Foglia v. Renal Ventures Management* ruling:

For reasons unrelated to the proper pleading standard required by Rule 9(b) in a False Claims Act case, the Solicitor General did not recommend granting certiorari in United States ex rel. Noah Nathan, even though the Solicitor General argued that the incorrect standard had been applied by the Fourth Circuit. Id.

THE FOLLOWING IS the Solicitor General's Brief submitted to the U.S. Supreme Court, edited, so it is easier to read for the non-lawyer. (The original unedited version is at the end of the chapter)

No. 12-1349

In the Supreme Court of the United States
UNITED STATES EX REL. NOAH NATHAN, PETITIONER
v.
TAKEDA PHARMACEUTICALS NORTH AMERICA, INC., ET AL.
ON PETITION FOR A WRIT OF CERTIORARI TO THE UNITED STATES COURT OF APPEALS FOR THE FOURTH CIRCUIT
BRIEF FOR THE UNITED STATES AS AMICUS CURIAE
DONALD B. VERRILLI, JR.
Solicitor General Counsel of Record
STUART F. DELERY
Assistant Attorney General
MALCOLM L. STEWART
Deputy Solicitor General
BRIAN H. FLETCHER
Assistant to the Solicitor General
MICHAEL S. RAAB
JOSHUA WALDMAN

Attorneys

Department of Justice Washington, D.C. 20530-0001 Supreme-CtBriefs@usdoj.gov (202) 514-2217

QUESTION PRESENTED

Whether a relator in a qui tam action under the False Claims Act, must identify specific false claims submitted for payment in order to plead fraud with sufficient particularity to satisfy Federal Rule of Civil Procedure 9(b).

(I have omitted the Table of Contents and the other cases referenced to keep it easier to read)

In the Supreme Court of the United States

No. 12-1349

UNITED STATES EX REL. NOAH NATHAN, PETITIONER

v.

TAKEDA PHARMACEUTICALS NORTH AMERICA, INC., ET AL.

ON PETITION FOR A WRIT OF CERTIORARI TO THE UNITED STATES COURT OF APPEALS FOR THE FOURTH CIRCUIT

BRIEF FOR THE UNITED STATES AS AMICUS CURIAE INTEREST OF THE UNITED STATES

This brief is submitted in response to the order of the Court inviting the Solicitor General to express the views of the United

States. In the view of the United States, the petition for a writ of certiorari should be denied.

STATEMENT

The False Claims Act (FCA), provides for the imposition of civil penalties and treble damages against any person who, "knowingly presents, or causes to be presented, a false or fraudulent claim for payment or approval." The "claims" subject to the FCA include "any request or demand for money or property" that is "presented to an officer, employee, or agent of the United States," as well as certain claims presented to entities that receive federal funds. The Attorney General may bring a civil action if he finds that a person has violated the FCA. Alternatively, a private person (known as a relator) may bring his own suit (commonly referred to as a qui tam action) "for the person and for the United States Government."

If a relator brings a qui tam action, the complaint is initially filed under seal and served upon the government, together with "substantially all material evidence and information the relator possesses." "The Government may elect to intervene and proceed with the action within 60 days after it receives both the complaint and the material evidence and information," and the district court may extend the 60-day period upon a showing of good cause. If the government declines to intervene, the relator "shall have the right to conduct the action," but the district court "may nevertheless permit the Government to intervene at a later date upon a showing of good cause." If a qui tam action results in the recovery of damages or civil penalties, the award is divided between the government and the relator.

This qui tam action alleges that a pharmaceutical company caused false claims to be presented to the federal Medicare and Medicaid programs by promoting one of its drugs for uses that have not been approved by the Food and Drug Administration (FDA).

Under the Federal Food, Drug, and Cosmetic Act (FDCA), a new drug may not be introduced into interstate commerce unless FDA has approved a new drug application based on the agency's determination that the drug is safe and effective for its intended use. FDA must also approve the drug's labeling, which specifies the FDA-approved uses and dosages for the drug.

Because a drug that is safe and effective for one use may be neither safe nor effective for others, FDA approval extends only to the uses specified in a drug's approved application and labeling. A new drug that is distributed for an intended use that has not been approved by FDA is "misbranded," and the FDCA prohibits its distribution in interstate commerce. A drug's "intended uses" are determined by the objective intent of the drug manufacturer, which may be demonstrated by the drug's "advertising" and by other "oral or written statements" by the manufacturer or its representatives. Accordingly, a manufacturer's promotion of a drug for unapproved uses may constitute evidence that the manufacturer has violated the FDCA's misbranding provisions by distributing a drug for an intended use that has not been approved by FDA.

FDA does not, however, attempt to regulate the practice of medicine. Once a drug is approved for one use at one dosage, doctors are free to prescribe it for unapproved uses or at other dosages—a practice that is sometimes called "off-label" prescribing.

Although prescriptions for unapproved uses are not prohibited by the FDCA, they may be ineligible for reimbursement under the federal Medicare and Medicaid programs. "Medicare is a federally funded health insurance program for the elderly and disabled." Medicaid is a cooperative federal- state program that funds medical care for needy individuals. Both programs provide coverage for certain prescription drugs. To be eligible for reimbursement, however, a drug generally must be prescribed for an FDA- approved use or for another "medically accepted indication" listed in one of several statutorily specified compendia.

Petitioner Noah Nathan is a sales manager employed by respondent Takeda Pharmaceuticals. Respondent manufacturers and sells a drug known as Kapidex, which suppresses the production of stomach acid. FDA has approved Kapidex for three indications: (1) for the healing of erosive esophagitis (EE), a condition in which refluxed stomach acid causes ulcers in the throat, with a recommended dose of 60 milligrams daily; (2) for the maintenance of healed EE, with a recommended dose of 30 milligrams daily; and (3) for the treatment of non-erosive gastroesophageal reflux disease (GERD), commonly known as heartburn or acid reflux, with a recommended dose of 30 milligrams daily. Petitioner alleged that the relevant compendia do not specify any other medically accepted indications for Kapidex, and that these three FDA-approved uses are therefore the only ones eligible for reimbursement under Medicare and Medicaid.

Petitioner contended that respondent had violated the FCA by knowingly causing Kapidex prescriptions written for unapproved uses to be presented to Medicare and Medicaid for reimbursement. Specifically, petitioner alleged that respondent had urged doctors to prescribe 60-milligram doses of Kapidex to GERD patients because respondent believed that a 60- milligram dose was more effective in treating GERD than the 30-milligram dose specified in the FDA- approved labeling. For example, petitioner alleged that respondent had offered samples of Kapidex exclusively in the 60-milligram dose and had provided those samples to primary care physicians and other doctors who treat GERD but generally do not treat active EE, the only condition for which a 60-milligram dose is approved. Petitioner alleged that respondent's actions had caused doctors to write prescriptions for unapproved uses; that some of those prescriptions had gone to patients covered by Medicare and Medicaid; and that false claims had resulted when those patients or their health care providers sought reimbursement from the federal health care programs.

Petitioner filed his qui tam complaint in September 2009. The government declined to intervene, and petitioner amended his complaint twice after it was unsealed. The district court dismissed the complaint without prejudice, finding it deficient in several respects. Petitioner then filed a third amended complaint, which the district court dismissed with prejudice on two alternative grounds.

The district court first held that the complaint failed to satisfy Federal Rule of Civil Procedure 9(b), which provides that a complaint alleging fraud "must state with particularity the circumstances constituting fraud." The court noted that petitioner's complaint "failed to identify any specific instances in which respondent caused a pharmacist or other healthcare provider to submit a claim for reimbursement to the government based on a non- reimbursable prescription." Instead, the complaint relied on "a combination of statistics and general allegations."

The district court held that this "statistics-based" approach failed to satisfy Rule 9(b). In particular, the court rejected petitioner's reliance on 98 Kapidex prescriptions written by 16 primary care physicians. Petitioner's complaint identified the 16 doctors by name, listed the month in which each prescription was written, and further alleged that each of the 98 prescriptions was submitted to Medicare for reimbursement. Petitioner did not, however, "allege that the prescriptions issued were in fact for 60 milligram doses." Instead, petitioner argued that it was reasonable to infer that more than 90% of the 98 prescriptions were for 60-milligram doses because the 16 doctors had received 60-milligram samples of Kapidex, and because more than 90% of respondent's overall sales of Kapidex are at the 60-milligram dose. The district court rejected that inference as too speculative, concluding that petitioner had not "alleged any basis on which to assume that the overall level of 60 milligram doses, as a percentage of overall Kapidex sales, corresponds to the prescriptions that were actually issued by these 16 primary care physicians."

The district court also held, in the alternative, that petitioner's complaint lacked plausible allegations that respondent had "caused" the presentation of false claims within the meaning of Section 3729(a)(1)(A). The court concluded that, even if Kapidex prescriptions for unapproved uses were submitted to Medicare and Medicaid for reimbursement, petitioner had failed to plead facts supporting a plausible inference that those prescriptions were caused by respondent's actions rather than by the independent judgment of the prescribing physicians.

The court of appeals affirmed. The court held that petitioner's complaint did not satisfy Rule 9(b) and the plausibility standard set forth in Ashcroft v. Iqbal, because petitioner had "failed to plausibly allege that any false claims had been presented to the government for payment."

The court of appeals first addressed the pleading standards governing FCA complaints, which must satisfy Rule 9(b) and must "state a claim to relief that is plausible on its face." The court held that, because "liability under the Act attaches only to a claim actually presented to the government for payment," a relator must "plead plausible allegations of presentment." The court further held that, under both Rule 9(b) and "the general plausibility standard of Iqbal," "'some indicia of reliability' must be provided in the complaint to support the allegation that an actual false claim was presented to the government."

The court of appeals identified some prior judicial decisions holding that "Rule 9(b) can be satisfied in the absence of particularized allegations of specific false claims." In the view of the court below, those cases involved circumstances in which "specific allegations of the defendant's fraudulent conduct necessarily led to the plausible inference that false claims were presented to the government." The court concluded, however, that where the defendant's alleged conduct "could have led, but need not necessarily have led, to the submission of false claims, a relator must allege with particularity that specific false claims actually were presented to the government." The court of appeals added that, "to the extent that other cases apply a more relaxed construction of Rule 9(b)," the court "disagreed with that approach."

The court of appeals then applied this standard to petitioner's allegation that 16 primary care physicians had written 98 Kapidex prescriptions that were submitted to Medicare. The court explained that, al- though petitioner "alleged that these 98 claims were presented to the government for payment," he did not "plausibly allege that the prescriptions were written for off-label uses." The court of appeals rejected as too "speculative" petitioner's contention that, because more than 90% of all Kapidex prescriptions are for the 60-milligram dose, a comparable percentage of these 98 specific prescriptions likely were for that dose. The court also noted that, even if some of the 98 prescriptions had been for the 60-milligram dose, those prescriptions were not necessarily ineligible for reimbursement because they could have been written to treat active EE, a condition for which the 60-milligram dose is approved.

DISCUSSION

Although the disagreement is not as clearly defined as petitioner contends, lower courts have reached inconsistent conclusions about the precise manner in which a qui tam relator may satisfy the requirements of Rule 9(b). Several courts of appeals have correctly held that a qui tam complaint satisfies Rule 9(b) if it contains detailed allegations supporting a plausible inference that false claims were submitted to the government, even if the complaint does not identify specific requests for payment. Other decisions, however, have articulated a per se rule that a relator must plead the details of particular false claims—that is, the dates and contents of bills or other demands for payment—to overcome a motion to dismiss.

This per se rule is unsupported by Rule 9(b) and undermines the FCA's effectiveness as a tool to combat fraud against the United States. Indeed, even those circuits that initially endorsed the per se rule have issued subsequent decisions that appear to adopt a more nuanced approach. The disagreement among the circuits therefore may be capable of resolution without this Court's intervention. If that disagreement persists, however, this Court's review to clarify the applicable pleading standard may ultimately be warranted in an appropriate case.

This case, however, is not a suitable vehicle for resolving the question presented. The court below correctly held that petitioner's complaint failed to satisfy the requirements of both Rule 9(b) and Ashcroft v. Iqbal, because it did not plausibly allege that false claims were presented to the government. Because the complaint failed not merely for lack of specificity, but also for lack of plausibility, this suit could not go forward even under the pleading standard most favorable to relators. Particularly because the issue continues to percolate in the lower courts, this Court's consideration of the question presented should await a case in which it would be outcome-determinative.

The lower courts have reached conflicting results about the application of Rule 9(b) in the FCA context. Recent decisions, however, create some uncertainty about the extent of the disagreement.

Although a plaintiff "must state with particularity the circumstances constituting fraud," several courts of appeals have correctly recognized that pleading the details of a specific false claim presented to the government is not an indispensable requirement of a viable FCA complaint. Even at trial, "a plaintiff does not necessarily need the exact dollar amounts, billing numbers, or dates to prove to a preponderance that fraudulent bills were actually submitted." To demand those details to survive a motion to dismiss is "significantly more than any federal pleading rule contemplates." Accordingly, several courts have held that a relator's complaint satisfies Rule 9(b) if it "alleges particular details of a scheme to submit false claims paired with reliable indicia that lead to a strong inference that claims were actually submitted."

The First and Fourth Circuits have also declined to adopt a per se rule requiring relators to plead specific false claims. The First Circuit has held that where— as in this case—a qui tam complaint alleges that "the defendant induced third parties to file false claims with the government," the complaint can "satisfy Rule 9(b) by providing 'factual or statistical evidence to strengthen the inference of fraud beyond possibility' without necessarily providing details as to each false claim." In the decision below, the Fourth Circuit endorsed the results in Grubbs and Duxbury and indicated that a relator need not identify particular false claims when "specific allegations of the defendant's fraudulent conduct necessarily lead to the plausible inference that false claims were presented to the government."

By contrast, the Sixth, Eighth, Tenth, and Eleventh Circuits have issued decisions finding that particular qui tam complaints should be dismissed under Rule 9(b) because the relators failed to identify specific requests for payment. "We hold that pleading an actual false claim with particularity is an indispensable element of a complaint that alleges a FCA violation in compliance with Rule 9(b)," requiring a relator to plead "some representative examples" of false claims. Affirming dismissal of a complaint that failed "to identify any specific false claim", holding that a relator must plead a specific false claim to avoid dismissal.

These courts, however, have not consistently adhered to this rigid understanding of Rule 9(b). The Sixth Circuit recently left open the possibility "that the requirement that a relator identify an actual false claim may be relaxed when, even though the relator is unable to produce an actual billing or invoice, he or she has pled facts which support a strong inference that a claim was submitted." The Tenth Circuit has likewise stated that an FCA complaint "need only show the specifics of a fraudulent scheme and provide an adequate basis for a reasonable inference that false claims were submitted as part of that scheme." And both the Eighth and Eleventh Circuits have allowed qui tam complaints to proceed notwithstanding relators' failure to identify "specific fraudulent claims for payment submitted to the government."

The First Circuit, too, has shifted its approach to this question. In 2004, that court appeared to adopt a per se rule that "a relator must provide details that identify particular false claims for payment." But the court later narrowed that holding, making clear that specific false claims need not be identified when the relator alleges that "the defendant induced third parties to file false claims with the government."

The current extent of the disagreement among the lower courts is thus uncertain, and the courts of appeals that have previously articulated a per se rule requiring relators to plead the details of specific false claims may have retreated from a rigid application of that rule. There is, however, at least some continuing uncertainty as to whether a qui tam complaint satisfies Rule 9(b) if it contains detailed allegations giving rise to a reasonable inference that false claims were submitted to the government, but does not identify specific requests for payment.

As the government explained when the Court sought the views of the United States on another petition raising the same question, a rigid rule that such complaints are inadequate would hinder the ability of qui tam relators to perform the role that Congress intended them to play in the detection and remediation of fraud against the United States. Qui tam complaints are often filed by the defendants' current and former employees. Such relators may be privy to detailed information indicating that their employers are engaged in fraud against the United States, and may be well-positioned to provide valuable assistance to the government's anti-fraud efforts, even if they are not privy to the details of the defendants' billing activities.

In Lusby, for example, an engineer who had worked for a government contractor alleged that his former employer had falsely represented that its aircraft engines met the government's specifications. And in Grubbs, a physician alleged that other doctors at his hospital had sought to recruit him into a scheme to bill the government for services they had not provided. Both relators came forward with detailed, plausible allegations of fraud. Yet under a per se rule requiring qui tam complaints to identify specific false claims, both suits would have been dismissed because neither relator was familiar with the minutiae of his employer's billing. Because a prospective relator is unlikely to be privy to such details unless she "works in the defendant's accounting department," a rule demanding the details of specific false claims would "take a big bite out of qui tam litigation."

Subjecting qui tam relators to a per se rule requiring the identification of specific false claims is especially unwarranted because it attaches dispositive significance to the relator's awareness of details that in most instances are already known to the government. The government rarely if ever needs a relator's assistance to identify claims for payment that have been submitted to the United States. Rather, relators typically contribute to the government's enforcement efforts by bringing to light other information that shows those claims to be false. Requiring qui tam complaints to identify specific false claims thus would not meaningfully assist the government's enforcement efforts. To the contrary, the likely effect of such a requirement would be to discourage the filing of qui tam suits by relators —like those in Grubbs and Lusby —who would otherwise have the means and the incentive to expose frauds against the United States.

The proper application of Rule 9(b) in the FCA context is thus a significant issue. If one or more courts of appeals continue to adhere to the rigid view that petitioner attributes to the court below, this Court's intervention may be warranted in a case where application of that approach appears to be outcome-determinative. This case, however, is not a suitable vehicle in which to take up the question. The court below correctly held that petitioner's complaint failed to satisfy Rule 9(b) and Iqbal because it does not plausibly allege that false claims were presented to the government. Petitioner's suit therefore could not go forward under the pleading standard adopted by any court of appeals.

Petitioner contends that the court of appeals found his complaint insufficient only because that court adopted an inflexible rule requiring qui tam relators to identify specific false claims. But the court of appeals did not adopt that per se rule. To the contrary, it required only "'some indicia of reliability' to support the allegation that an actual false claim was presented to the government." The court stated that a relator must identify specific false claims only where the "defendant's actions, as alleged and as reasonably inferred from the allegations, could have led, but need not necessarily have led, to the submission of false claims." Although this articulation of the pleading standard differs from the phrasing used by other circuits, it does not require that every qui tam complaint plead the details of specific false claims.

Petitioner contends that, by requiring a relator to identify specific false claims whenever a defendant's conduct would not "necessarily" have led to the submission of false claims, the court of appeals improperly elevated Iqbal's plausibility requirement to a demand that relators "prove falsity." But the court below did not require such proof; rather, it rejected petitioner's complaint because petitioner had failed to "plausibly allege" the presentation of false claims. The court of appeals explained, moreover, that a relator's complaint is sufficient if the defendant's actions "as alleged and as reasonably inferred from the allegations" would "necessarily have led to the submission of false claims."

That formulation suggests that petitioner's complaint would have satisfied the court's standard if petitioner had alleged facts sufficient to support a reasonable inference that false claims were submitted.

The court of appeals' rejection of a per se rule is further confirmed by the balance of its opinion. If the court had followed the decisions demanding that a relator plead "representative examples" of specific false claims, or the "dates, times, or amounts of individual false claims," it would have rejected petitioner's complaint out of hand, because there is no dispute that petitioner failed to allege the details of any request for payment made to the federal government. (Petitioner provided some details concerning 98 Kapidex prescriptions, including the names of the prescribing doctors and the months in which the prescriptions were written. He also generally alleged that all 98 prescriptions were submitted to Medicare for reimbursement.) He provided no dates, amounts, or other details, however, about the circumstances under which reimbursement was sought. Despite the conceded absence of any allegation of a specific false claim, however, the court of appeals carefully examined the complaint to determine whether it provided a plausible basis for inferring that false claims were presented. And as to the 98 Kapidex prescriptions on which petitioner now relies, the court's analysis indicates that its decision rested chiefly on the complaint's lack of plausibility, not its lack of particularity. The court characterized petitioner's allegation regarding those 98 prescriptions as resting on "speculative" and "implausible" assertions, and the court framed its holding as a conclusion that petitioner had not "plausibly alleged that the 98 prescriptions were written for off- label uses."

This lack of plausible allegations that respondent's conduct led to the presentation of false claims would have doomed petitioner's complaint before every court of appeals, even those that apply the most relator- friendly pleading standards (requiring "factual or statistical evidence to strengthen the inference of fraud beyond possibility") (complaint need not "exclude all possibility of honesty," but must contain more than "vague and unsubstantiated allegations of fraud"); (requiring "reliable indicia that lead to a strong inference that claims were actually submitted"). Because the deficiencies in petitioner's complaint would have resulted in dismissal in any circuit, the disagreement about the application of Rule 9(b) in FCA cases is not implicated here.

Petitioner contends that the court of appeals was wrong to find his allegations implausible. But the question whether this particular complaint plausibly alleged the presentation of false claims to the government is a factbound issue that would not warrant this Court's review even if the court of appeals had erred. In any event, the decision below is correct.

Petitioner relies on the allegation that 16 primary care physicians wrote 98 Kapidex prescriptions that were ultimately submitted to Medicare for reimbursement. Petitioner did not, however, directly allege that those prescriptions were ineligible for reimbursement. Instead, petitioner argues that general allegations and nationwide statistics about Kapidex prescriptions support an inference that these 98 prescriptions were for 60-milligram rather than 30- milligram doses, and a further inference that the prescriptions were for GERD rather than for the healing of active EE (an indication for which a 60-milligram dose is approved). As the court of appeals correctly held, the allegations in petitioner's complaint do not support either inference.

First, the complaint does not provide a plausible basis for inferring that the 98 prescriptions were for 60-milligram doses. Petitioner contends that "there is a 'more than 90%' certainty" that these prescriptions were for 60-milligram doses because the 16 doctors received 60-milligram samples and because 93% of all Kapidex prescriptions are written for 60- milligram doses. As the court of appeals observed, however, the complaint fails to "connect these general statistics to the 98 prescriptions identified."

Although petitioner's theory of the case assumes that these 98 prescriptions were representative of Kapidex prescriptions nationwide, "it is logical to assume that a much lower-than-average percentage of the 98 prescriptions were written for 60 mg doses" given the complaint's allegation that primary care physicians generally "do not treat the condition for which the higher 60 mg dose is indicated."

Second, the complaint does not provide a plausible basis for inferring that the 98 prescriptions were written to treat GERD rather than EE. Petitioner alleged that, in general, primary care physicians "do not regularly treat EE." But he did not allege that primary care physicians never treat EE, and he also did not allege anything about the patient populations or practices of the 16 specific primary care physicians who wrote the prescriptions at issue here.

As the First Circuit explained in rejecting an analogous FCA action against a manufacturer that had allegedly marketed one of its drugs for unapproved uses, "it is a possible but not a necessary or even strong inference that doctors" wrote prescriptions for Kapidex for unapproved uses and that "some false claims for Kapidex reimbursement were submitted to the government" as a result. Like the complaint in Rost, petitioner's pleading "contained no factual or statistical evidence to strengthen the inference of fraud beyond possibility." Accordingly, petitioner's suit would fail under the pleading standard adopted by any court of appeals.

It is also unclear whether petitioner's complaint would ultimately survive respondent's motion to dismiss even if this Court granted certiorari and reversed the court of appeals' judgment. The district court dismissed petitioner's complaint on the independent ground that petitioner had failed adequately to plead causation. The court of appeals found it unnecessary to address that alternative holding. Even if this Court granted certiorari and held that petitioner had pleaded facts sufficient to create an inference that false claims were submitted, petitioner's suit could not go forward if the court of appeals on remand were to agree with the district court on the issue of causation.

THE PETITION for a writ of certiorari should be denied. Respectfully submitted.

FEBRUARY 2014
DONALD B. VERRILLI, JR.
Solicitor General
STUART F. DELERY
Assistant Attorney General
MALCOLM L. STEWART
Deputy Solicitor General
BRIAN H. FLETCHER
Assistant to the Solicitor General
MICHAEL S. RAAB
JOSHUA WALDMAN
Attorneys

FEBRUARY 2014

HERE IS the original unedited version

No. 12-1349
In the Supreme Court of the United States
UNITED STATES EX REL. NOAH NATHAN, PETITIONER
v.
TAKEDA PHARMACEUTICALS NORTH AMERICA, INC., ET AL.
ON PETITION FOR A WRIT OF CERTIORARI TO THE

UNITED STATES COURT OF APPEALS FOR THE FOURTH CIRCUIT

BRIEF FOR THE UNITED STATES AS AMICUS CURIAE
DONALD B. VERRILLI, JR.
Solicitor General Counsel of Record
STUART F. DELERY
Assistant Attorney General
MALCOLM L. STEWART
Deputy Solicitor General
BRIAN H. FLETCHER
Assistant to the Solicitor General
MICHAEL S. RAAB
JOSHUA WALDMAN
Attorneys

DEPARTMENT OF JUSTICE WASHINGTON, D.C. 20530-0001 Supreme-CtBriefs@usdoj.gov (202) 514-2217

QUESTION PRESENTED

Whether a relator in a qui tam action under the False Claims Act, 31 U.S.C. 3729 et seq., must identify specific false claims submitted for payment in order to plead fraud with sufficient particularity to satisfy Federal Rule of Civil Procedure 9(b).

TABLE OF CONTENTS

Interest of the United States
Statement
Discussion Conclusion

TABLE OF AUTHORITIES:

Arkansas Dep't of Health & Human Servs. v. Ahlborn
Ashcroft v. Iqbal,
Baycol Prods. Litig.,
Buckman Co. v. Plaintiffs' Legal Comm.
Chesbrough v. VPA, P.C.
Ebeid v. Lungwitz,
Hopper v. Solvay Pharm., Inc
Thomas Jefferson Univ. v. Shalala,
United States ex rel. Bledsoe v. Community Health
Sys., Inc.,
United States ex rel. Clausen v. Laboratory Corp. of
Am.
United States ex rel. Duxbury v. Ortho Biotech
Prods., L.P.,
United States ex rel. Eisenstein v. City of N.Y.,
United States ex rel. Grubbs v. Kanneganti,
United States ex rel. Joshi v. St. Luke's Hosp., Inc.,
United States ex rel. Karvelas v. Melrose-Wakefield
Hosp.,
United States ex rel. Lemmon v. Envirocare of Utah,
Inc.,
United States ex rel. Lusby v. Rolls-Royce Corp.,
United States ex rel. Rost v. Pfizer, Inc.,
United States ex rel. Sikkenga v. Regence BlueCross
BlueShield
United States ex rel. Walker v. R&F Props. of Lake
Cnty., Inc.
Washington Legal Found. v. Henney

Statutes, regulations and rule:
False Claims Act, 31 U.S.C. 3729 et seq.:
U.S.C. 3729(a)(1)(A)
U.S.C. 3729(b)(2)

U.S.C. 3730(a)

U.S.C. 3730(b)(1)

U.S.C. 3730(b)(2)

U.S.C. 3730(b)(3)

U.S.C. 3730(c)(3)

U.S.C. 3730(d)

Federal Food, Drug, and Cosmetic Act, 21 U.S.C. 301 et seq.:

U.S.C. 331(a)

U.S.C. 352(f)

U.S.C. 355(a)

U.S.C. 355(b)(1)(F)

U.S.C. 355(d)

Fraud Enforcement and Recovery Act of 2009,

Pub. L. No. 111-21, § 4(a), 123 Stat. 1621

U.S.C. 1395w-102 (2006 & Supp. V 2011)

U.S.C. 1395w-102(e)(1) (2006 & Supp. V 2011)

U.S.C. 1395w-102(e)(4) (Supp. V 2011)

U.S.C. 1396b(i)(10)

U.S.C. 1396r-8 (2006 & Supp. V 2011)

U.S.C. 1396r-8(g)(1)(B)(i).

U.S.C. 1396r-8(k)(3)

U.S.C. 1396r-8(k)(6)

C.F.R.:

Section 201.5

Section 201.5(b)

Section 201.55-201.57

Section 201.128

Fed. R. Civ. P. 9(b)

In the Supreme Court of the United States

No. 12-1349

UNITED STATES EX REL. NOAH NATHAN, PETITIONER

v.

TAKEDA PHARMACEUTICALS NORTH AMERICA, INC., ET AL.

ON PETITION FOR A WRIT OF CERTIORARI TO THE UNITED STATES COURT OF APPEALS FOR THE FOURTH CIRCUIT

BRIEF FOR THE UNITED STATES AS AMICUS CURIAE INTEREST OF THE UNITED STATES

THIS BRIEF IS SUBMITTED in response to the order of the Court inviting the Solicitor General to express the views of the United States. In the view of the United States, the petition for a writ of certiorari should be denied.

STATEMENT

1. The False Claims Act (FCA), 31 U.S.C. 3729 et seq., provides for the imposition of civil penalties and treble damages against any person who, inter alia, "knowingly presents, or causes to be presented, a false or fraudulent claim for payment or approval." 31 U.S.C. 3729(a)(1)(A). The "claims" subject to the FCA include "any request or demand * * * for money or property" that is "presented to an officer, employee, or agent of the United States," as well as certain claims presented to entities that receive federal funds. 31 U.S.C. 3729(b)(2).1 The Attorney General may bring a civil action if he finds that a person has violated the FCA. 31 U.S.C. 3730(a). Alternatively, a private person (known as a relator) may bring his own suit (commonly referred to as a qui tam action) "for the person and for the United States Government." 31 U.S.C. 3730(b)(1); see United States ex rel. Eisenstein v. City of New York, 556 U.S. 928, 930 (2009).

If a relator brings a qui tam action, the complaint is initially filed under seal and served upon the government, together with "substantially all material evidence and information the [relator] possesses." 31 U.S.C. 3730(b)(2). "The Government may elect to intervene and proceed with the action within 60 days after it receives both the complaint and the material evidence and information," ibid., and the district court may extend the 60-day period upon a showing of good cause, 31 U.S.C. 3730(b)(3). If the government de- clines to intervene, the relator "shall have the right to conduct the action," but the district court "may nevertheless permit the Government to intervene at a later date upon a showing of good cause." 31 U.S.C. 3730(c)(3). If a qui tam action results in the recovery of damages or civil penalties, the award is divided between the government and the relator. 31 U.S.C. 3730(d).

---

1 Section 3729 was amended while the conduct at issue in this case was ongoing. See Fraud Enforcement and Recovery Act of 2009, Pub. L. No. 111-21, § 4(a), 123 Stat. 1621. The changes are not material to the question presented, and the parties and the courts below appear to have agreed that the amended statute governs this case. See Pet. App. 2a, 24a.

2. This qui tam action alleges that a pharmaceutical company caused false claims to be presented to the federal Medicare and Medicaid programs by promoting one of its drugs for uses that have not been approved by the Food and Drug Administration (FDA).

a. Under the Federal Food, Drug, and Cosmetic Act (FDCA), 21 U.S.C. 301 et seq., a new drug may not be introduced into interstate commerce unless FDA has approved a new drug application based on the agency's determination that the drug is safe and effective for its intended use. 21 U.S.C. 355(a) and (d). FDA must also approve the drug's labeling, which specifies, inter alia, the FDA-approved uses and dos- ages for the drug. 21 U.S.C. 355(b)(1)(F) and (d); 21 C.F.R. 201.5(b), 201.55-201.57.

Because a drug that is safe and effective for one use may be neither safe nor effective for others, FDA approval extends only to the uses specified in a drug's approved application and labeling. 21 U.S.C. 355(d). A new drug that is distributed for an intended use that has not been approved by FDA is "misbranded," and the FDCA prohibits its distribution in interstate commerce. 21 U.S.C. 352(f); 21 C.F.R. 201.5; see 21 U.S.C. 331(a). A drug's "intended uses" are deter- mined by the objective intent of the drug manufacturer, which may be demonstrated by the drug's "advertising" and by other "oral or written statements" by the manufacturer or its representatives. 21 C.F.R. 201.128. Accordingly, a manufacturer's promotion of a drug for unapproved uses may constitute evidence that the manufacturer has violated the FDCA's misbranding provisions by distributing a drug for an intended use that has not been approved by FDA. See Washington Legal Found. v. Henney, 202 F.3d 331, 332-333 (D.C. Cir. 2000).

FDA does not, however, attempt to regulate the practice of medicine. Once a drug is approved for one use at one dosage, doctors are free to prescribe it for unapproved uses or at other dosages—a practice that is sometimes called "off-label" prescribing. See 59 Fed. Reg. 59,820, 59,821 (Nov. 18, 1994); Washington Legal Found., 202 F.3d at 332-333; cf. Buckman Co. v. Plaintiffs' Legal Comm., 531 U.S. 341, 350-351 (2001) (discussing the similar statutory scheme governing medical devices).

b. Although prescriptions for unapproved uses are not prohibited by the FDCA, they may be ineligible for reimbursement under the federal Medicare and Medicaid programs. "Medicare is a federally funded health insurance program for the elderly and disabled." Thomas Jefferson Univ. v. Shalala, 512 U.S. 504, 506 (1994). Medicaid is a cooperative federal- state program that funds medical care for needy individuals. Arkansas Dep't of Health & Human Servs. v. Ahlborn, 547 U.S. 268, 275 (2006). Both programs provide coverage for certain prescription drugs. See 42 U.S.C. 1395w-102 (2006 & Supp. V 2011) (Medicare); 42 U.S.C. 1396r-8 (2006 & Supp. V 2011) (Medicaid). To be eligible for reimbursement, however, a drug generally must be prescribed for an

FDA- approved use or for another "medically accepted indication" listed in one of several statutorily specified compendia. 42 U.S.C. 1395w-102(e)(1) (2006 & Supp. V 2011); 42 U.S.C. 1395w-102(e)(4) (Supp. V 2011); 42 U.S.C. 1396b(i)(10), 1396r-8(k)(3) and (6); see 42 U.S.C. 1396r-8(g)(1)(B)(i) (identifying compendia).

c. Petitioner Noah Nathan is a sales manager employed by respondent Takeda Pharmaceuticals. Pet. App. 2a. Respondent manufacturers and sells a drug known as Kapidex, which suppresses the production of stomach acid. Id. at 3a.2 FDA has approved Kapidex for three indications: (1) for the healing of erosive esophagitis (EE), a condition in which refluxed stomach acid causes ulcers in the throat, with a recommended dose of 60 milligrams daily; (2) for the maintenance of healed EE, with a recommended dose of 30 milligrams daily; and (3) for the treatment of non-erosive gastroesophageal reflux disease (GERD), commonly known as heartburn or acid reflux, with a recommended dose of 30 milligrams daily. Id. at 4a. Petitioner alleged that the relevant compendia do not specify any other medically accepted indications for Kapidex, and that these three FDA-approved uses are therefore the only ones eligible for reimbursement under Medicare and Medicaid. Id. at 77a.

Petitioner contended that respondent had violated the FCA by knowingly causing Kapidex prescriptions written for unapproved uses to be presented to Medicare and Medicaid for reimbursement. Specifically, petitioner alleged that respondent had urged doctors to prescribe 60-milligram doses of Kapidex to GERD patients because respondent believed that a 60- milligram dose was more effective in treating GERD than the 30-milligram dose specified in the FDA- approved labeling. Pet. App. 3a-4a. For example, petitioner alleged that respondent had offered samples of Kapidex exclusively in the 60-milligram dose and had provided those samples to primary care physicians and other doctors who treat GERD but generally do not treat active EE, the only condition for which a 60-milligram dose is approved. Id. at

4a. Petitioner alleged that respondent's actions had caused doctors to write prescriptions for unapproved uses; that some of those prescriptions had gone to patients covered by Medicare and Medicaid; and that false claims had resulted when those patients or their health care providers sought reimbursement from the federal health care programs. Id. at 41a, 44a-45a.

2 Kapidex is now known as "Dexilant." Pet. App. 3a n.3. Like the decisions below, this brief refers to the drug as Kapidex.

3. Petitioner filed his qui tam complaint in September 2009. The government declined to intervene, and petitioner amended his complaint twice after it was unsealed. The district court dismissed the complaint without prejudice, finding it deficient in several respects. Pet. App. 17a-18a & n.10. Petitioner then filed a third amended complaint, which the district court dismissed with prejudice on two alternative grounds. Id. at 19a-31a.

a. The district court first held that the complaint failed to satisfy Federal Rule of Civil Procedure 9(b), which provides that a complaint alleging fraud "must state with particularity the circumstances constituting fraud." See Pet. App. 22a-28a. The court noted that petitioner's complaint "failed to identify any specific instances in which [respondent] caused a pharmacist or other healthcare provider to submit a claim for reimbursement to the government based on a non- reimbursable prescription." Id. at 24a. Instead, the complaint relied on "a combination of statistics and general allegations." Ibid.

The district court held that this "statistics-based" approach failed to satisfy Rule 9(b). Pet. App. 24a. In particular, the court rejected petitioner's reliance on 98 Kapidex prescriptions written by 16 primary care physicians. Petitioner's complaint identified the 16 doctors by name, listed the month in which each prescription was written, and further alleged that each of the 98 prescriptions was submitted to Medicare for reimbursement. Id. at 26a-27a; see id. at 105a-109a. Petitioner did not, however, "allege that the prescriptions issued were in fact for 60 milligram doses." Id.

at 26a. Instead, petitioner argued that it was reasonable to infer that more than 90% of the 98 prescriptions were for 60-milligram doses because the 16 doctors had received 60-milligram samples of Kapidex, and because more than 90% of respondent's overall sales of Kapidex are at the 60-milligram dose. Ibid. The district court rejected that inference as too speculative, concluding that petitioner had not "allege[d] any basis on which to assume that the overall level of 60 milligram doses, as a percentage of overall Kapidex sales, corresponds to the prescriptions that were actually issued by these [16] primary care physicians." Id at 26a-27a.3

b. The district court also held, in the alternative, that petitioner's complaint lacked plausible allegations that respondent had "caused" the presentation of false claims within the meaning of Section 3729(a)(1)(A). Pet. App. 28a-29a. The court concluded that, even if Kapidex prescriptions for unapproved uses were submitted to Medicare and Medicaid for reimbursement, petitioner had failed to plead facts supporting a plausible inference that those prescriptions were caused by respondent's actions rather than by the independent judgment of the prescribing physicians. Id. at 29a.

3 In the lower courts, petitioner unsuccessfully argued that other, more general allegations in his complaint independently satisfied Rule 9(b). Pet. App. 11a-16a, 24a-28a. His petition for certiorari, however, relies only on the 98 prescriptions written by 16 primary care physicians. See Pet. 9-10, 30-31.

4. The court of appeals affirmed. Pet. App. 1a-18a. The court held that petitioner's complaint did not satisfy Rule 9(b) and the plausibility standard set forth in Ashcroft v. Iqbal, 556 U.S. 662, 678 (2009), because petitioner had "failed to plausibly allege that any false claims had been presented to the government for payment." Pet. App. 2a.

The court of appeals first addressed the pleading standards governing FCA complaints, which must satisfy Rule 9(b) and must "state a claim to relief that is plausible on its face," Iqbal, 556

U.S. at 678. See Pet. App. 5a-6a. The court held that, because "liability under the Act attaches only to a claim actually presented to the government for payment," a relator must "plead plausible allegations of presentment." Id. at 8a. The court further held that, under both Rule 9(b) and "the general plausibility standard of Iqbal," "'some indicia of reliability' must be provided in the complaint to support the allegation that an actual false claim was presented to the government." Id. at 8a-9a (quoting United States ex rel. Clausen v. Laboratory Corp. of Am., 290 F.3d 1301, 1311 (11th Cir. 2002), cert. denied, 537 U.S. 1105 (2003)).

The court of appeals identified some prior judicial decisions holding that "Rule 9(b) can be satisfied in the absence of particularized allegations of specific false claims." Pet. App. 9a. In the view of the court below, those cases involved circumstances in which "specific allegations of the defendant's fraudulent conduct necessarily led to the plausible inference that false claims were presented to the government." Id. at 9a-10a (citing United States ex rel. Grubbs v. Kanneganti, 565 F.3d 180, 192 (5th Cir. 2009); United States ex rel. Duxbury v. Ortho Biotech Prods., L.P., 579 F.3d 13, 30 (1st Cir. 2009), cert. denied, 130 S. Ct. 3454 (2010)). The court concluded, however, that where the defendant's alleged conduct "could have led, but need not necessarily have led, to the submission of false claims, a relator must allege with particularity that specific false claims actually were present- ed to the government." Id. at 10a. The court of appeals added that, "[t]o the extent that other cases apply a more relaxed construction of Rule 9(b)," the court "disagree[d] with that approach." Ibid.

The court of appeals then applied this standard to petitioner's allegation that 16 primary care physicians had written 98 Kapidex prescriptions that were submitted to Medicare. The court explained that, al- though petitioner "allege[d] that these [98] claims were presented to the government for payment," he did not "plausibly allege that the prescriptions were written for off-label uses." Pet. App. 13a. The court of appeals rejected as too "speculative" petitioner's contention that, because more than 90% of all Kapidex prescriptions are for the 60-milligram dose, a comparable percentage of these 98 specific prescriptions likely were for that dose. Id. at 13a-14a. The court also noted that, even if some of the 98 prescriptions had been for the 60-milligram dose, those prescriptions were not necessarily ineligible for reimbursement because they could have been written to treat active EE, a condition for which the 60-milligram dose is approved. Id. at 14a.4

DISCUSSION

Although the disagreement is not as clearly defined as petitioner contends, lower courts have reached inconsistent conclusions about the precise manner in which a qui tam relator may satisfy the requirements of Rule 9(b). Several courts of appeals have correctly held that a qui tam complaint satisfies Rule 9(b) if it contains detailed allegations supporting a plausible inference that false claims were submitted to the government, even if the complaint does not identify specific requests for payment. Other decisions, however, have articulated a per se rule that a relator must plead the details of particular false claims—that is, the dates and contents of bills or other demands for payment—to overcome a motion to dismiss.

This per se rule is unsupported by Rule 9(b) and undermines the FCA's effectiveness as a tool to combat fraud against the United States. Indeed, even those circuits that initially endorsed the per se rule have issued subsequent decisions that appear to adopt a more nuanced approach. The disagreement among the circuits therefore may be capable of resolution without this Court's intervention. If that disagreement persists, however, this Court's review to clarify the applicable pleading standard may ultimately be warranted in an appropriate case.

4 Because it affirmed the dismissal of petitioner's complaint based on the failure to plausibly allege that false claims were presented to the government, the court of appeals did not

consider the district court's alternative holding that petitioner had failed adequately to allege causation. Pet. App. 5a.

This case, however, is not a suitable vehicle for resolving the question presented. The court below correctly held that petitioner's complaint failed to satisfy the requirements of both Rule 9(b) and Ashcroft v. Iqbal, 556 U.S. 662 (2009), because it did not plausibly allege that false claims were presented to the government. Because the complaint failed not merely for lack of specificity, but also for lack of plausibility, this suit could not go forward even under the pleading standard most favorable to relators. Particularly because the issue continues to percolate in the lower courts, this Court's consideration of the question presented should await a case in which it would be outcome-determinative.

1. The lower courts have reached conflicting results about the application of Rule 9(b) in the FCA context. Recent decisions, however, create some uncertainty about the extent of the disagreement.

a. Although a plaintiff "must state with particularity the circumstances constituting fraud," Fed. R. Civ. P. 9(b), several courts of appeals have correctly recognized that pleading the details of a specific false claim presented to the government is not an indispensable requirement of a viable FCA complaint. Even at trial, "a plaintiff does not necessarily need the exact dollar amounts, billing numbers, or dates to prove to a preponderance that fraudulent bills were actually submitted." United States ex rel. Grubbs v. Kanneganti, 565 F.3d 180, 190 (5th Cir. 2009). To demand those details to survive a motion to dismiss is "significantly more than any federal pleading rule contemplates." Ibid. Accordingly, several courts have held that a relator's complaint satisfies Rule 9(b) if it "alleg[es] particular details of a scheme to submit false claims paired with reliable indicia that lead to a strong inference that claims were actually submitted." Ibid.; see Ebeid v. Lungwitz, 616 F.3d 993, 998-999 (9th Cir.) (same), cert. denied, 131 S. Ct. 801 (2010); United States ex rel. Lusby v. Rolls-

Royce Corp., 570 F.3d 849, 854 (7th Cir. 2009) (Easterbrook, C.J.) ("We don't think it essential for a relator to produce the invoices (and accompanying representations) at the outset of the suit.").

The First and Fourth Circuits have also declined to adopt a per se rule requiring relators to plead specific false claims. The First Circuit has held that where— as in this case—a qui tam complaint alleges that "the defendant induced third parties to file false claims with the government," the complaint can "satisfy Rule 9(b) by providing 'factual or statistical evidence to strengthen the inference of fraud beyond possibility' without necessarily providing details as to each false claim." United States ex rel. Duxbury v. Ortho Bio- tech Prods., L.P., 579 F.3d 13, 29 (2009) (quoting United States ex rel. Rost v. Pfizer, Inc., 507 F.3d 720, 733 (1st Cir. 2007)), cert. denied 130 S. Ct. 3454 (2010). In the decision below, the Fourth Circuit endorsed the results in Grubbs and Duxbury and indicated that a relator need not identify particular false claims when "specific allegations of the defendant's fraudulent conduct necessarily [lead] to the plausible inference that false claims were presented to the government." Pet. App. 9a.

b. By contrast, the Sixth, Eighth, Tenth, and Eleventh Circuits have issued decisions finding that particular qui tam complaints should be dismissed under Rule 9(b) because the relators failed to identify specific requests for payment. See, e.g., United States ex rel. Bledsoe v. Community Health Sys., Inc., 501 F.3d 493, 504 (6th Cir. 2007) ("We hold that pleading an actual false claim with particularity is an indispensable element of a complaint that alleges a FCA violation in compliance with Rule 9(b)."); United States ex rel. Joshi v. St. Luke's Hosp., Inc., 441 F.3d 552, 560 (8th Cir.) (requiring a relator to plead "some representative examples" of false claims), cert. denied, 549 U.S. 881 (2006); United States ex rel. Sikkenga v. Regence BlueCross BlueShield, 472 F.3d 702, 727-728 (10th Cir. 2006) (affirming dismissal of a complaint that failed "to identify any specific [false] claim"); Hopper v. Solvay Pharm.,

Inc., 588 F.3d 1318, 1326 (11th Cir. 2009) (holding that a relator must plead a specific false claim to avoid dismissal), cert. denied, 130 S. Ct. 3465 (2010).

These courts, however, have not consistently adhered to this rigid understanding of Rule 9(b). The Sixth Circuit recently left open the possibility "that the requirement that a relator identify an actual false claim may be relaxed when, even though the relator is unable to produce an actual billing or invoice, he or she has pled facts which support a strong inference that a claim was submitted." Chesbrough v. VPA, P.C., 655 F.3d 461, 471 (2011). The Tenth Circuit has likewise stated that an FCA complaint "need only show the specifics of a fraudulent scheme and provide an adequate basis for a reasonable inference that false claims were submitted as part of that scheme." Unit- ed States ex rel. Lemmon v. Envirocare of Utah, Inc., 614 F.3d 1163, 1172 (2010) (citing Duxbury, 579 F.3d at 29; Lusby, 570 F.3d at 854-855; Grubbs, 565 F.3d at 190). And both the Eighth and Eleventh Circuits have allowed qui tam complaints to proceed notwithstanding relators' failure to identify "specific fraudulent claims for payment submitted to the government." In re Baycol Prods. Litig., 732 F.3d 869, 875-877 (8th Cir. 2013); see United States ex rel. Walker v. R&F Props. of Lake Cnty., Inc., 433 F.3d 1349, 1360 (11th Cir. 2005), cert. denied, 549 U.S. 1027 (2006); see also United States ex rel. Clausen v. Laboratory Corp. of Am., 290 F.3d 1301, 1311 (11th Cir. 2002) (stating that a qui tam complaint must contain "some indicia of reliability * * * to support the allegation of an actual false claim for payment") (emphasis omitted), cert. denied, 537 U.S. 1105 (2003).5

c. The current extent of the disagreement among the lower courts is thus uncertain, and the courts of appeals that have previously articulated a per se rule requiring relators to plead the details of specific false claims may have retreated from a rigid application of that rule. There is, however, at least some contin- uing uncertainty as to whether a qui tam complaint satisfies Rule

9(b) if it contains detailed allegations giving rise to a reasonable inference that false claims were submitted to the government, but does not identify specific requests for payment.

As the government explained when the Court sought the views of the United States on another petition raising the same question, a rigid rule that

---

5 The First Circuit, too, has shifted its approach to this question. In 2004, that court appeared to adopt a per se rule that "a relator must provide details that identify particular false claims for payment." United States ex rel. Karvelas v. Melrose-Wakefield Hosp., 360 F.3d 220, 232, cert. denied, 543 U.S. 820 (2004). But the court later narrowed that holding, making clear that specific false claims need not be identified when the relator alleges that "the defendant induced third parties to file false claims with the government." Duxbury, 579 F.3d at 29. such complaints are inadequate would hinder the ability of qui tam relators to perform the role that Congress intended them to play in the detection and remediation of fraud against the United States. See U.S. Amicus Br. at 16-17, Ortho Biotech Prods., L.P. v. United States ex rel. Duxbury, No. 09-654 (May 19, 2010). Qui tam complaints are often filed by the defendants' current and former employees. Such relators may be privy to detailed information indicating that their employers are engaged in fraud against the United States, and may be well-positioned to provide valuable assistance to the government's anti-fraud efforts, even if they are not privy to the details of the defendants' billing activities.

In Lusby, for example, an engineer who had worked for a government contractor alleged that his former employer had falsely represented that its aircraft engines met the government's specifications. See 570 F.3d at 853-854. And in Grubbs, a physician alleged that other doctors at his hospital had sought to recruit him into a scheme to bill the government for services they had not provided. See 565 F.3d at 191- 192. Both relators came forward with detailed, plausible allegations of fraud. Yet under a per se rule requiring qui tam complaints to identify specific false claims, both suits would have been dismissed because neither relator was familiar with the minutiae of his employer's billing. Because a prospective relator is unlikely to be privy to such details unless she "works in the defendant's accounting department," a rule demanding the details of specific false claims would "take[] a big bite out of qui tam litigation." Lusby, 570 F.3d at 854.

Subjecting qui tam relators to a per se rule requiring the identification of specific false claims is especially unwarranted because it attaches dispositive significance to the relator's awareness of details that in most instances are already known to the government. The government rarely if ever needs a relator's assistance to identify claims for payment that have been submitted to the United States. Rather, relators typically contribute to the government's enforcement efforts by bringing to light other information that shows those claims to be false. Requiring qui tam complaints to identify specific false claims thus would not meaningfully assist the government's enforcement efforts. To the contrary, the likely effect of such a requirement would be to discourage the filing of qui tam suits by relators —like those in Grubbs and Lusby —who would otherwise have the means and the incentive to expose frauds against the United States.

2. The proper application of Rule 9(b) in the FCA context is thus a significant issue. If one or more courts of appeals continue to adhere to the rigid view that petitioner attributes to the court below (but see pp. 13-14, supra), this Court's intervention may be warranted in a case where application of that approach appears to be outcome-determinative. This case, however, is not a suitable vehicle in which to take up the question. The court below correctly held that petitioner's complaint failed to satisfy Rule 9(b) and Iqbal because it does not plausibly allege that false claims were presented to the government. Petitioner's suit there-

fore could not go forward under the pleading standard adopted by any court of appeals.

a. Petitioner contends (Pet. 19-20; Reply Br. 3-4 & n.2) that the court of appeals found his complaint insufficient only because that court adopted an inflexible rule requiring qui tam relators to identify specific false claims. But the court of appeals did not adopt that per se rule. To the contrary, it required only "'some indicia of reliability' * * * to support the allegation that an actual false claim was presented to the government." Pet. App. 8a (quoting Clausen, 290 F.3d at 1311). The court stated that a relator must identify specific false claims only where the "defend- ant's actions, as alleged and as reasonably inferred from the allega- tions, could have led, but need not necessarily have led, to the submission of false claims." Id. at 10a. Although this articulation of the pleading standard differs from the phrasing used by other circuits, it does not require that every qui tam complaint plead the details of specific false claims.6

The court of appeals' rejection of a per se rule is further confirmed by the balance of its opinion. If the court had followed the decisions demanding that a relator plead "representative examples" of specific false claims, Joshi, 441 F.3d at 557, or the

---

6 Petitioner contends (Reply Br. 5) that, by requiring a relator to identify specific false claims whenever a defendant's conduct would not "necessarily" have led to the submission of false claims, the court of appeals improperly elevated Iqbal's plausibility requirement to a demand that relators "prov[e] falsity." But the court below did not require such proof; rather, it rejected petitioner's complaint because petitioner had failed to "plausibly allege" the presentation of false claims. Pet. App. 2a, 13a. The court of appeals explained, moreover, that a relator's complaint is sufficient if the defendant's actions "as alleged and as reasonably inferred from the allegations" would "necessarily have led[] to the submission of false claims." Id. at 10a (emphasis altered). That

formulation suggests that petitioner's complaint would have satisfied the court's standard if petitioner had alleged facts sufficient to support a reasonable inference that false claims were submitted.

"DATES, times, or amounts of individual false claims," Hopper, 588 F.3d at 1326, it would have rejected petitioner's complaint out of hand, because there is no dispute that petitioner failed to allege the details of any request for payment made to the federal government. See Pet. 29-30.7 Despite the conceded absence of any allegation of a specific false claim, however, the court of appeals carefully examined the complaint to determine whether it provided a plausible basis for inferring that false claims were presented. Pet. App. 11a- 17a. And as to the 98 Kapidex prescriptions on which petitioner now relies, the court's analysis indicates that its decision rested chiefly on the complaint's lack of plausibility, not its lack of particularity. The court characterized petitioner's allegation regarding those 98 prescriptions as resting on "speculative" and "implausible" assertions, and the court framed its holding as a conclusion that petitioner had not "plausibly allege[d] that the [98] prescriptions were written for off- label uses." Id. at 13a-14a.

This lack of plausible allegations that respondent's conduct led to the presentation of false claims would have doomed petitioner's complaint before every court of appeals, even those that apply the most relator- friendly pleading standards. See, e.g., Duxbury, 579 F.3d at 29 (requiring "factual or statistical evidence to strengthen the inference of fraud beyond

---

7 Petitioner provided some details concerning 98 Kapidex prescriptions, including the names of the prescribing doctors and the months in which the prescriptions were written. Pet. App. 105a- 109a. He also generally alleged that all 98 prescriptions were

submitted to Medicare for reimbursement. Ibid. He provided no dates, amounts, or other details, however, about the circumstances under which reimbursement was sought. See ibid. possibility" (quoting Rost, 507 F.3d at 733)); Lusby, 570 F.3d at 854-855 (complaint need not "exclude all possibility of honesty," but must contain more than "vague and unsubstantiated allegations of fraud"); Grubbs, 565 F.3d at 190 (requiring "reliable indicia that lead to a strong inference that claims were actually submitted"); Ebeid, 616 F.3d at 998-999 (same). Because the deficiencies in petitioner's complaint would have resulted in dismissal in any circuit, the disagreement about the application of Rule 9(b) in FCA cases is not implicated here.

b. Petitioner contends (Pet. 28-33) that the court of appeals was wrong to find his allegations implausible. But the question whether this particular complaint plausibly alleged the presentation of false claims to the government is a factbound issue that would not warrant this Court's review even if the court of appeals had erred. In any event, the decision below is correct.

Petitioner relies on the allegation that 16 primary care physicians wrote 98 Kapidex prescriptions that were ultimately submitted to Medicare for reimbursement. Petitioner did not, however, directly allege that those prescriptions were ineligible for reimbursement. Instead, petitioner argues that general allegations and nationwide statistics about Kapidex prescriptions support an inference that these 98 prescriptions were for 60-milligram rather than 30- milligram doses, and a further inference that the prescriptions were for GERD rather than for the healing of active EE (an indication for which a 60-milligram dose is approved). As the court of appeals correctly held, the allegations in petitioner's complaint do not support either inference.

First, the complaint does not provide a plausible basis for inferring that the 98 prescriptions were for 60-milligram doses. Petitioner contends (Pet. 31) that "there is a 'more than 90%' certainty" that these prescriptions were for 60-milligram doses because the 16 doctors received 60-milligram samples and because 93% of all Kapidex prescriptions are written for 60-milligram doses. As the court of appeals observed, however, the complaint fails to "connect[] these general statistics to the 98 prescriptions identified." Pet. App. 14a. Although petitioner's theory of the case assumes that these 98 prescriptions were representative of Kapidex prescriptions nationwide, "it is logical to assume that a much lower-than-average percentage of the 98 prescriptions were written for 60 mg doses" given the complaint's allegation that primary care physicians generally "do not treat the condition for which the higher 60 mg dose is indicated." Ibid.

Second, the complaint does not provide a plausible basis for inferring that the 98 prescriptions were written to treat GERD rather than EE. Pet. App. 14a-15a. Petitioner alleged that, in general, primary care physicians "do not regularly treat EE." Id. at 84a. But he did not allege that primary care physicians never treat EE, and he also did not allege any- thing about the patient populations or practices of the 16 specific primary care physicians who wrote the prescriptions at issue here. Id. at 14a.

As the First Circuit explained in rejecting an analogous FCA action against a manufacturer that had allegedly marketed one of its drugs for unapproved uses, "it is a possible but not a necessary or even strong inference that doctors" wrote prescriptions for Kapidex for unapproved uses and that "some false claims for [Kapidex] reimbursement were submitted to the government" as a result. Rost, 507 F.3d at 732. Like the complaint in Rost, petitioner's pleading "contained no factual or statistical evidence to strengthen the inference of fraud beyond possibility." Id. at 733. Accordingly, petitioner's suit would fail under the pleading standard adopted by any court of appeals.8

---

8 It is also unclear whether petitioner's complaint would ultimately survive respondent's motion to dismiss even if this Court granted certiorari and reversed the court of appeals' judgment.

The district court dismissed petitioner's complaint on the independent ground that petitioner had failed adequately to plead causation. Pet. App. 28a-29a. The court of appeals found it unnecessary to address that alternative holding. See id. at 5a; note 4, supra. Even if this Court granted certiorari and held that petitioner had pleaded facts sufficient to create an inference that false claims were submitted, petitioner's suit could not go forward if the court of appeals on remand were to agree with the district court on the issue of causation.

THE PETITION for a writ of certiorari should be denied. Respectfully submitted.

FEBRUARY 2014
DONALD B. VERRILLI, JR.
Solicitor General
STUART F. DELERY
Assistant Attorney General
MALCOLM L. STEWART
Deputy Solicitor General
BRIAN H. FLETCHER
Assistant to the Solicitor General
MICHAEL S. RAAB
JOSHUA WALDMAN
Attorneys

FEBRUARY 2014

20

FOGLIA V. RENAL VENTURES MGMT., LLC.

The case *Foglia v. Renal Ventures Mgmt., Llc.*, was argued in the Federal 3rd Circuit Court of Appeals shortly after my case was denied by the U.S. Supreme Court. Foglia was decided on June 6, 2014, and had the opportunity to use the Solicitor General's Brief to the U.S. Supreme Court regarding my case from February 2014. Foglia was argued September 11, 2013, but the court included in their decision the Solicitor General's Brief which was written five months after the argument.

THE ENTIRE DECISION is at the end of the chapter but I want to point out the court's ruling in relation to my case. I will edit the following to make it easier to read but the entire decision at the end of the chapter will remain unedited.

II.

Before we are able to decide whether Foglia has met the higher pleading requirements set by Federal Rule of Civil Procedure 9(b), and so whether he has stated a claim under Federal

Rule of Civil Procedure 12(b)(6), we must first determine what Rule 9(b) requires of an FCA claimant, an issue this court has not had occasion to rule on specifically. Rule 9(b) states, "in alleging fraud or mistake, a party must state with particularity the circumstances constituting fraud or mistake. Malice, intent, knowledge, and other conditions of a person's mind may be alleged generally." However, the various Circuits disagree as to what a plaintiff, such as Foglia, must show at the pleading stage to satisfy the "particularity" requirement of Rule 9(b) in the context of a claim under the FCA.

The Fourth, Sixth, Eighth, and Eleventh Circuits have held that a plaintiff must show "representative samples" of the alleged fraudulent conduct, specifying the time, place, and content of the acts and the identity of the actors. See United States ex rel. Noah Nathan v. Takeda Pharm. N. Am., Inc., The First, Fifth, and Ninth Circuits, however, have taken a more nuanced reading of the heightened pleading requirements of Rule 9(b), holding that it is sufficient for a plaintiff to allege "particular details of a scheme to submit false claims paired with reliable indicia that lead to a strong inference that claims were actually submitted."

In United States ex Rel. Wilkins v. United Health Group, Inc., we noted that we had never "held that a plaintiff must identify a specific claim for payment at the pleading stage of the case to state a claim for relief." While that conclusion does not itself commit us to the more nuanced standards favored by the First, Fifth, and Ninth Circuits, it is hard to reconcile the text of the FCA, which does not require that the exact content of the false claims in question be shown, with the "representative samples" standard favored by the Fourth, Sixth, Eighth, and Eleventh Circuits. As the Fifth Circuit has stated, requiring this sort of detail at the pleading stage would be "one small step shy of requiring production of actual documentation with the complaint, a level of proof not demanded to win at trial and significantly more than any federal pleading rule contemplates."

Furthermore, in a recent brief for the United States as amicus curiae, filed in relation to the petition for a writ of certiorari in United States ex rel. Noah Nathan, a case presenting a factual situation similar to that presented here, the Solicitor General indicated that the United States also believes that the heightened or "rigid" pleading standard required by the Fourth, Sixth, Eighth, and Eleventh Circuits is "unsupported by Rule 9(b) and undermines the FCA's effectiveness as a tool to combat fraud against the United States." The Solicitor General's brief further states that "pleading the details of a specific false claim presented to the government is not an indispensable requirement of a viable FCA complaint." Brief for the United States as Amicus Curiae, United States ex rel Noah Nathan v. Takeda Pharm. N. Am., Inc., 2014. The Solicitor General also noted that even the Circuits which purport to follow the "rigid understanding of Rule 9(b)" have "not consistently adhered" to it, providing a further ground for doubting whether the "rigid" understanding of Rule 9(b) could be the correct one. Insofar as the purpose of Rule 9(b) is to "provide defendants with fair notice of the plaintiffs' claims," the more "nuanced" approach followed by the First, Fifth, and Ninth Circuits will suffice. That standard is also compatible with our earlier ruling in Wilkins, and we will use that standard in this case.

For reasons unrelated to the proper pleading standard required by Rule 9(b) in a FCA case, the Solicitor General did not recommend granting certiorari in United States ex rel. Noah Nathan, even though the Solicitor General argued that the incorrect standard had been applied by the Fourth Circuit. Id.

Foglia mentioned that the Solicitor General did not recommend that the U.S. Supreme Court take my case. In my opinion, with the conservative makeup of the court at the time, there was a concern that if they did accept my case, and rule against me, then the entire country would be bad for whistleblowers by having to adhere to the "strict pleading standard" interpretation of the Rule 9(b) as set by the Fourth Circuit.

THE ORIGINAL RULING

UNITED STATES COURT OF APPEALS FOR THE THIRD CIRCUIT ______

No. 12-4050 ________

THOMAS FOGLIA,

In the Name of the United States Government pursuant to the False Claims Act, 31 U.S.C. Section 3730; the State of New Jersey False Claims Act, Title 2A of the New Jersey Statutes and Amending 3 P.L. 1968, C. 413; The State of Texas pursuant to TEX.HUM.RES.CODE Sect. 36.001-26.117 and individually pursuant to the New Jersey Conscientious Employee Protection Act, N.J.S.A. 34:19-1 et Seq.

Appellant

v.

RENAL VENTURES MANAGEMENT, LLC _______

On Appeal from the United States District Court for the District of New Jersey

(D.C. No. 1-09-cv-01552)

District Judge: Honorable Noel L. Hillman ______

Argued: September 11, 2013

MCKEE, CHIEF JUDGE, SMITH, and SLOVITER, Circuit Judges (Filed: June 6, 2014)

PRECEDENTIAL

Ross Begelman, Esquire (Argued) Marc M. Orlow, Esquire Begelman, Orlow & Melletz

411 Route 70 East

Suite 245

Cherry Hill, NJ 08034

Counsel for Appellant

R. James Kravitz, Esquire

Barry J. Muller, Esquire (Argued)

Fox Rothchild

997 Lenox Drive

Princeton Pike Corporate Center, Building 3 Lawrenceville, NJ 08648

Counsel for Appellee

———————

OPINION ——————

SLOVITER, Circuit Judge.

Thomas Foglia appeals the District Court's order dismissing his qui tam claim brought under the False Claims Act, 31 U.S.C. § 3729 et. seq. Foglia's complaint arises out of claims submitted or presented to Medicare by Defendant Renal Ventures ("Renal") that Foglia alleges are fraudulent. The District Court dismissed on the ground that the complaint failed to state a claim.1

1 The District Court had jurisdiction over Relator Foglia's federal claims pursuant to 28 U.S.C. § 1331, and over Relator's related state law claim under 28 U.S.C. § 1367. We have jurisdiction pursuant to 28 U.S.C. § 1291. We review de novo a district court's grant of a motion to dismiss for failure to state a claim under Federal Rule of Civil Procedure 12(b)(6). See Jordan v. Fox, Rothschild, O'Brien & Frankel, 20 F.3d 1250, 1261 (3d Cir. 1994). We "are required to accept as true all allegations in the complaint and all reasonable inferences that can be drawn from them after construing them in the light most favorable to the non- movant." Id. (citations omitted)

I.

Foglia is a registered nurse who was employed with Renal starting on March 13, 2007, and was terminated around November 7, 2008. (App. 34) Renal is a dialysis care services company. (App. 34) Foglia filed a qui tam complaint against Renal on behalf of himself as a relator and on behalf of the United States under the False Claims Act ("FCA") in April 2009. (App. 25) The United States chose not to intervene. (App. 25) Foglia filed an amended complaint, and the District Court granted Renal's motion for judgment on the pleadings and gave Foglia twenty days to file a second amended complaint. (App. 67, 29) It was Foglia's second amended complaint ("SAC") that was before the District Court in the proceeding below. (App. 33)

In the argument before us, counsel for Foglia described his claim as in two parts; one was certification and the other was retaliation.2 He claimed that Renal violated the FCA by falsely certifying that it was in compliance with state regulations regarding quality of care, by falsely submitting claims for reimbursement for the drug Zemplar, and by reusing single-use Zemplar vials. (App. 50-56) The District Court granted Renal's Motion to Dismiss the FCA complaint under Federal Rule of Civil Procedure 12(b)(6) because it determined that Foglia had failed to state his claim with the heightened level of particularity required by Federal Rule of Civil Procedure 9(b) for fraud claims. (App. 12-13) In particular, the District Court focused on Foglia's failure to provide a "representative sample" (App. 12) or to "identify representative examples of specific false claims made to the Government." (App. 16) The District Court also determined that even if Foglia's claim had met the requirement of Rule 9(b), Foglia "provided no authority under an express or implied false certification theory that the claims submitted by defendant violated a rule or statute establishing compliance as a condition of payment." (App. 16) The District Court dismissed the SAC with prejudice, stating that it did so in light of the fact that Foglia had twice amended his complaint and had engaged in initial discovery. (App. 22) Foglia here appeals the dismissal of his claim in relation to over-billing on Zemplar.

2 The retaliation claim was not considered by the District Court and is not relevant to this appeal. Foglia also sued under the New Jersey False Claims Act for the same violations and brought suit under the New Jersey Conscientious Employee Protection Act. (App. 56-58) Because Renal had not moved to dismiss Foglia's state law claims, the District Court chose not to exercise supplemental jurisdiction over these claims and dismissed them without prejudice. We therefore need not consider them here.

II.

Before we are able to decide whether Foglia has met the higher pleading requirements set by Federal Rule of Civil Procedure 9(b), and so whether he has stated a claim under Federal Rule of Civil Procedure 12(b)(6), we must first determine what Rule 9(b) requires of an FCA claimant, an issue this court has not had occasion to rule on specifically. Rule 9(b) states, "[i]n alleging fraud or mistake, a party must state with particularity the circumstances constituting fraud or mistake. Malice, intent, knowledge, and other conditions of a person's mind may be alleged generally." Fed. R. Civ. P. 9(b). However, the various Circuits disagree as to what a plaintiff, such as Foglia, must show at the pleading stage to satisfy the "particularity" requirement of Rule 9(b) in the context of a claim under the FCA.

The Fourth, Sixth, Eighth, and Eleventh Circuits have held that a plaintiff must show "representative samples" of the alleged fraudulent conduct, specifying the time, place, and content of the acts and the identity of the actors. See United States ex rel. Noah Nathan v. Takeda Pharm. N. Am., Inc., 707 F.3d 451, 455-56 (4th Cir. 2013), cert. denied, 2014 WL 1271321 (U.S. Mar. 31, 2014) (No. 12-1349); United States ex rel. Bledsoe v. Cmty. Health Sys., Inc., 501

F.3d 493, 510 (6th Cir. 2007); United States ex rel. Joshi v. St. Luke's Hosp., Inc., 441 F.3d 552, 557 (8th Cir. 2006); United States ex rel. Clausen v. Lab. Corp. of Am., Inc., 290 F.3d 1301, 1308, 1312 (11th Cir. 2002). The First,3 Fifth, and Ninth Circuits, however, have taken a more nuanced reading of the heightened pleading requirements of Rule 9(b), holding that it is sufficient for a plaintiff to allege "particular details of a scheme to submit false claims paired with reliable indicia that lead to a strong inference that claims were actually submitted." United States ex rel. Grubbs v. Kanneganti, 565 F.3d 180, 190 (5th Cir. 2009); see also Ebeid ex rel. United States v. Lungwitz, 616 F.3d 993, 998-99 (9th Cir. 2010).

In United States ex Rel. Wilkins v. United Health Group, Inc., 659 F.3d 295, 308 (3d Cir. 2011), we noted that we had never "held that a plaintiff must identify a specific claim for payment at the pleading stage of the case to state a claim for relief." (Emphasis in the original, citation omitted). While that conclusion does not itself commit us to the more nuanced standards favored by the First, Fifth, and Ninth Circuits, it is hard to reconcile the text of the FCA, which does not require that the exact content of the false claims in question be shown, with the "representative samples" standard favored by the Fourth, Sixth, Eighth, and Eleventh Circuits. As the Fifth Circuit has stated, requiring this sort of detail at the pleading stage would be "one small step shy of requiring production of actual documentation with the complaint, a level of proof not demanded to win at trial and significantly more than any federal pleading rule contemplates." Grubb, 565 F.3d at 190 (citations and footnote omitted).

Furthermore, in a recent brief for the United States as amicus curiae, filed in relation to the petition for a writ of certiorari in United States ex rel. Noah Nathan, 707 F.3d 451, a case presenting a factual situation similar to that presented here, the Solicitor General indicated that the United States also believes that the heightened or "rigid" pleading standard required by the Fourth, Sixth, Eighth, and Eleventh Circuits is "unsupported by Rule 9(b) and undermines the FCA's effectiveness as a tool to combat fraud against the United States." The Solicitor General's brief further states that "pleading the details of a specific false claim presented to the government is not an indispensable requirement of a viable FCA complaint." Brief for the United States as Amicus Curiae at 10-11, United States ex rel Noah Nathan v. Takeda Pharm. N. Am., Inc., 2014 WL 1271321 (U.S. Mar. 31, 2014) (No. 12-1249), denying cert. to 707 F.3d 451. The Solicitor General also noted that even the Circuits which purport to follow the "rigid understanding of Rule 9(b)" have "not consistently adhered" to it, id. at 13, providing a further ground for doubting whether the "rigid" understanding of Rule 9(b) could be the correct one. 4 Insofar as the purpose of Rule 9(b) is to "provide[] defendants with fair notice of the plaintiffs' claims," id., the more "nuanced"5 approach followed by the First, Fifth, and Ninth Circuits will suffice. That standard is also compatible with our earlier ruling in Wilkins, and we will use that standard in this case.

3 THE FIRST CIRCUIT previously held the more restrictive view. See United States ex rel. Karvelas v. Melrose-Wakefield Hosp., 360 F.3d 220, 226 (1st Cir. 2004), but has recently moved to a more relaxed approach much closer to that followed by the Fifth Circuit. See United States ex rel. Duxbury v. Ortho Biotech Prods., L.P., 579 F.3d 13, 29 (1st Cir. 2009).

4 For reasons unrelated to the proper pleading standard required by Rule 9(b) in a FCA case, the Solicitor General did not recommend granting certiorari in United States ex rel. Noah Nathan, even though the Solicitor General argued that the incorrect standard had been applied by the Fourth Circuit. Id.

5 The Solicitor General's brief uses this construction, and we find it appropriate.

· · ·

III.

We thus turn to the question of whether Foglia has met the requirements of Rule 9(b) as set out above. Although not presented as clearly as it might be, Foglia's "overfill" claim is best understood as a "factually false" claim. "A claim is factually false when the claimant misrepresents what goods or services that it provided to the Government." Wilkins, 659 F.3d at 305. Foglia contends that Renal over-charged the government for Zemplar, a prescription drug used for the prevention and treatment of secondary hyperparathyroidism associated with chronic kidney disease. Zemplar comes in vials of three sizes, but Renal only uses 5 microgram ("mcg") vials. The vials were originally designed to be single-use only, with any unused medicine (characterized, somewhat misleadingly, as "overfill" by Foglia6) discarded. When Zemplar vials are used in this single-use fashion, Medicare is charged for the full content of the vial, no matter how much of the content is actually used. Foglia contends that Renal charged Medicare as if Renal were using the 5 mcg vials in the recommended "single use" fashion, when in fact it harvested unused portions from vials and used this harvested amount on other patients. (App. 47-48)

Originally, the Department of Health and Human Services ("HSS") required that Zemplar always be used in a single use fashion. However, in September of 2002 (several years before the alleged false claim in this case), HSS issued a memorandum allowing for the multiple use of individual Zemplar vials and other injectable medicines if six conditions were followed, so as to ensure the safe use of the medicine. (App. 60)7 Foglia contends that Renal "continued multiple use of single use vials of injectable medications such as Zemplar consistently without regard to complying with the conditions set forth by HHS." (App. 47) Because we are at the complaint stage in the proceedings we must accept as true all allegations in the complaint, and therefore must accept the allegation that Renal did not, in fact, comply with the required recommendations by HHS for the safe re-use of Zemplar vials.

In order for Foglia to satisfy the standards of Rule 9(b), as we have adopted them here, he must provide "particular details of a scheme to submit false claims paired with reliable indicia that lead to a strong inference that claims were actually submitted." See Grubbs, 565 F.3d at 190. Describing a mere opportunity for fraud will not suffice. Sufficient facts to establish "a plausible ground for relief" must be alleged. Fowler v. UPMC Shadyside, 578 F.3d 203, 211 (3d Cir. 2009) (internal citation omitted). While not presented as clearly as it might be, the essentials of Foglia's factually false claim argument seem to be as follows. Inventory logs maintained by Renal show that, during the month of October 2008, Renal used from 29 to 35 vials of Zemplar per day. (App. 75-6) Because Renal orders Zemplar in only 5 mcg vials (App. 48), it would have needed 50 vials of Zemplar each of the days in question for the number of patients actually seen each day, if the 5 mcg vials were used in the single use fashion. (App. 76) Foglia contends that because renal was using only 29-35 vials of Zemplar per day, it must have been harvesting unused Zemplar from previously used vials. However, these allegations are not enough to establish a "strong inference" that false claims were submitted, as the use of harvested "extra" Zemplar is permitted if the HHS recommendations noted above are followed, and it is therefore possible that Renal was not over-charging.

We are therefore faced with two possible scenarios. Either, as Foglia alleges, Renal was charging the government as if it were using vials of Zemplar in the single use fashion while actually harvesting and using "extra" Zemplar from the vials, or Renal was using the "extra" Zemplar from bottles and only charging the government for the actual volume of Zemplar used, despite not being in compliance with the regulations for using Zemplar in this fashion. While both scenarios are possible, it is unclear what would motivate the second, as it would expose Renal to possible sanctions for failure to comply with required procedures, and would not provide any financial incentive.

This is a close case as to meeting the requirements of Rule 9(b). Accepting the factual assertions made by Foglia as true, we have patient logs that show that less Zemplar was used than would be required if it were used in the single use fashion. We know that Medicare will reimburse for the full vial of Zemplar, regardless of whether all of the Zemplar is used, and that this provides an opportunity for the sort of fraud alleged by Foglia. At this point we must assume that Foglia is correct in alleging that Renal did not follow the procedures that it should have followed if it was to harvest the "extra" Zemplar from the used vials. Although we recognize that this hypothesis could be challenged, it certainly suffices to give Renal notice of the charges against it, as is required by Rule 9(b). This conclusion is further supported by the fact that Renal, and only Renal, has access to the documents that could easily prove the claim one way or another—the full billing records from the time under consideration. Under these circumstances, Foglia has provided sufficient facts to meet the requirements under Rule 9(b), and has therefore also met the requirements to state a claim under 12(b)(6).

6 PUT MOST ACCURATELY, "OVERFILL" is the "extra" amount of a medicine in a vial which is always included so as to ensure that a full dose of the labeled amount for the vial is possible, despite any incidental waste. For example, when, only 2 mcgs of a 5 mcg vial are used, the remaining 3 mcgs are not strictly "overfill." The name used here is not important, however. What matters is the claim that Renal was harvesting "extra" Zemplar from already-used vials to administer to patients.

7 Foglia, in his brief and in his SAC, styles these conditions as "express 'conditions for receiving payment'." (App. 46) Though

we have not directly ruled on the issue, it is highly doubtful these conditions for safe use are properly "conditions for receiving payment." Cf. Mikes v. Straus, 274 F.3d 687, 699 (2d Cir. 2001) ("the False Claims Act was not designed for use as a blunt instrument to enforce compliance with all medical regulations—but rather only those regulations that are a precondition of payment.") However, while this would be relevant for a "legally false" claim argument, Foglia seems to have abandoned this argument, and the "conditions for receiving payment" aspect is not directly relevant for a "factually false" claim argument.

IV.

For the foregoing reasons, we will reverse the dismissal of the factually false claim portion of Foglia's SAC and remand to the District Court for further appropriate proceedings in accordance with this opinion.

CASES REFERRING TO NATHAN V. TAKEDA

Some important cases have been given their own chapters in this book, but I also wanted to include some other current noteworthy litigation concerning Rule 9(b) as well.

As in other chapters, I will edit the legal writing to make it easier for the non-lawyer while providing the unedited version at the end of the chapter.

The American Health Lawyers Association[1] shows "the rationale of the Solicitor General's briefing in Takeda has been persuasive to courts who are being asked whether Rule 9(b) requires qui tam relators to plead specific examples of allegedly false claims. For example, in June of this year, the D.C. Circuit rejected a defense argument that Rule 9(b) requires a relator to plead "representative examples" of the false claims. In doing so, the court (quoting language from the Solicitor General's briefing in Takeda) stated that "the federal government itself already has records of those payments and thus 'rarely if ever needs a relator's assistance to identify claims for payment that have been submitted.'" The bottom line is that the proper application of Rule 9(b) continues to be hard-fought by litigants, and the Supreme Court will be called on again to resolve this question."

UNITED STATES EX REL. Campos v. Johns Hopkins Health Sys. Corp.,[2]"The heightened pleading standard plays a particularly important role in qui tam actions, where the plaintiff, "who has suffered no injury in fact, may be particularly likely to file suit as a pretext to uncover unknown wrongs." In light of this, the Fourth Circuit recently clarified that "when a defendant's actions, as alleged and as reasonably inferred from the allegations, could have led, but need not necessarily have led, to the submission of false claims, a relator must allege with particularity that specific false claims actually were presented to the government for payment." *United States ex rel. Nathan v. Takeda Pharmaceuticals North America, Inc.* The court ruled that, "Campos's complaint fails under *Takeda* because he alleges a scheme that need not necessarily have led to the submission of false claims and fails to identify particular false claims that were actually presented." "Recognizing that this may be a tough pill for such plaintiffs to swallow, the Fourth Circuit said the following:

In reaching this conclusion, we acknowledge the practical challenges that a relator may face in cases such as the present one, in which a relator may not have independent access to records such as prescription invoices, and where privacy laws may pose a barrier to obtaining such information without court involvement. Nevertheless, our pleading requirements do not permit a relator to bring an action without pleading facts that support all the elements of a claim. We further emphasize, however, that the standard we articulate today does not foreclose claims under the Act when a relator plausibly pleads that specific, identifiable claims actually were presented to the government for payment."

The court granted the defendants motion to dismiss.

United States Ex Rel. Ryan v. Endo Pharm., Inc.,[3] "The Circuits are split as to the degree of specificity required in alleging FCA claims. The Fourth, Sixth, Eighth and Eleventh Circuits require that a plaintiff must show "representative samples" of the "alleged fraudulent conduct, specifying time, place, and content of the acts and the identity of the actors." See *United States ex rel. Noah Nathan v. Takeda Pharm. N. Am., Inc.* The First, Fifth and Ninth Circuits have taken a slightly different approach holding that Rule 9(b) only requires a plaintiff to allege "particular details of a scheme to submit false claims paired with reliable indicia that lead to a strong inference that claims were actually submitted."

"Until recently, the Court of Appeals for the Third Circuit ("Third Circuit") had not entered the fray and declared the level of specificity required under Rule 9(b) in pleading an FCA qui tam action. However, recently in *Foglia v. Renal Ventures Mgmt., LLC,* the Third Circuit rejected the stricter standard applied by the Fourth, Sixth, Eighth and Eleventh Circuits reasoning that requiring "representative samples" would be "one small step shy of requiring production of actual documentation with the complaint, a level of proof not demanded to win at trial and significantly more than any federal pleading rule contemplates." Instead, the Court adopted the more lenient standard utilized in the First, Fifth and Ninth Circuits, finding that it adequately satisfies Rule 9(b)'s purpose of giving the defendants fair notice of the claims against it."

The court ruled in favor of the whistleblower which prompted Endo Pharmaceuticals into a settlement agreement with the government for $171.9 million.[4]

. . .

In U.S. ex rel. Palmieri et al v. Alpharma Inc. et al[5] in the U.S. District Court for the District of Maryland, the judge ruled against the relator Palmieri using my case as her justification. Judge Hollander stated, "Nathan is binding circuit precedent that is completely dispositive of the issue. It dictates that the amended complaint must be dismissed for failure to state a claim upon which relief can be granted." Concerning the information needed to proceed in the case Judge Hollander said, "by the nature of the scheme alleged, it is doubtful that such information would be in Mr. Palmieri's possession - the false claims themselves would have been submitted by patients, or at best by their physicians, but not by anyone in defendants' employ".[6] By the judge's statement, meaning that they are requiring information that a whistle-blower, as an employee of the company, could not gain access to, potentially gives a free pass to pharmaceutical companies due to HIPAA regulations.

THE FOLLOWING ARE the unedited versions.

THE AMERICAN HEALTH LAWYERS ASSOCIATION[7] shows "the rationale of the Solicitor General's briefing in Takeda has been persuasive to courts who are being asked whether Rule 9(b) requires qui tam relators to plead specific examples of allegedly false claims. For example, in June of this year, the D.C. Circuit rejected a defense argument that Rule 9(b) requires a relator to plead "representative examples" of the false claims. In doing so, the court (quoting language from the Solicitor General's briefing in Takeda) stated that "the federal government itself already has records of those payments and thus 'rarely if ever needs a relator's assistance to identify claims for payment that have been submitted.'" United States ex rel. Heath v. AT & T, Inc., No. 14-7094, 2015 WL 3852180, at *11 (D.C. Cir. June 23, 2015) (citation omitted). The bottom line is that the proper application of Rule 9(b) continues to be hard-fought by litigants, and the Supreme Court will be called on again to resolve this question."

UNITED STATES EX REL. *Campos v. Johns Hopkins Health Sys. Corp.,*[8] Civil No. CCB-17-2156 (D. Md. Apr. 24, 2018) ("The heightened pleading standard plays a particularly important role in qui tam actions, where the plaintiff, "who has suffered no injury in fact, may be particularly likely to file suit as a pretext to uncover unknown wrongs." Owens, 612 F.3d at 731-32 (internal citation and quotation marks omitted). In light of this, the Fourth Circuit recently clarified that "when a defendant's actions, as alleged and as reasonably inferred from the allegations, could have led, but need not necessarily have led, to the submission of false claims, a relator must allege with particularity that specific false claims actually were presented to the government for payment." *United States ex rel. Nathan v. Takeda Pharmaceuticals North America, Inc.,* 707 F.3d 451, 457 (4th Cir. 2013).")

UNITED STATES EX RE. *Ryan v. Endo Pharm., Inc.,*[9] 27 F.Supp.3d 615, 623-24 (E.D. Pa. 2014) ("The Circuits are split as to the degree of specificity required in alleging FCA claims. The Fourth, Sixth, Eighth and Eleventh Circuits require that a plaintiff must show "representative samples" of the "alleged fraudulent conduct, specifying time, place, and content of the acts and the identity of the actors." See *United States ex rel. Noah Nathan v. Takeda Pharm. N. Am., Inc.,* 707 F.3d 451, 455–56 (4th Cir.2013), cert. denied, ——— U.S. ———, 134 S.Ct. 1759, 188 L.Ed.2d 592 (2014) ; *United States ex rel. Bledsoe v. Cmty. Health Sys., Inc.,* 501 F.3d 493, 510 (6th Cir.2007) ; *United States ex rel. Joshi v. St. Luke's Hosp., Inc.,* 441 F.3d 552,

557 (8th Cir.2006) ; *United States ex rel. Clausen v. Lab. Corp. of Am., Inc.*, 290 F.3d 1301, 1308, 1312 (11th Cir.2002). The First, Fifth and Ninth Circuits have taken a slightly different approach holding that Rule 9(b) only requires a plaintiff to allege "particular details of a scheme to submit false claims paired with reliable indicia that lead to a strong inference that claims were actually submitted." *United States ex rel. Duxbury v. Ortho Biotech Prods., LP*, 579 F.3d 13, 29 (1st Cir.2009) ; *United States ex rel. Grubbs v. Kanneganti*, 565 F.3d 180, 190 (5th Cir.2009) ; *Ebeid ex rel. United States v. Lungwitz*, 616 F.3d 993, 998–99 (9th Cir.2010). Until recently, the Court of Appeals for the Third Circuit ("Third Circuit") had not entered the fray and declared the level of specificity required under Rule 9(b) in pleading an FCA qui tam action. See *United States ex rel. Underwood v. Genentech, Inc.*, 720 F.Supp.2d 671, 672 (E.D.Pa.2010) (noting the silence on the issue). However, recently in *Foglia v. Renal Ventures Mgmt., LLC*, 754 F.3d 153 (3d Cir.2014), the Third Circuit rejected the stricter standard applied by the Fourth, Sixth, Eighth and Eleventh Circuits reasoning that requiring "representative samples" would be "one small step shy of requiring production of actual documentation with the complaint, a level of proof not demanded to win at trial and significantly more than any federal pleading rule contemplates." 754 F.3d at 156 (quoting Grubbs, 565 F.3d at 190). Instead, the Court adopted the more lenient standard utilized in the First, Fifth and Ninth Circuits, finding that it adequately satisfies Rule 9(b)'s purpose of giving the defendants fair notice of the claims against it. See Id. at 156–57.")

In *U.S. ex rel. Palmieri et al v. Alpharma Inc. et al*[10] in the U.S. District Court for the District of Maryland, the judge ruled against the relator Palmieri using my case as her justification. Judge Hollander stated, "Nathan is binding circuit precedent that is completely dispositive of the issue. It dictates that the amended complaint must be dismissed for failure to state a claim upon which relief can be granted." Concerning the information needed to proceed in the case Judge Hollander said, "by the nature of the scheme alleged, it is doubtful that such information would be in Mr. Palmieri's possession - the false claims themselves would have been submitted by patients, or at best by their physicians, but not by anyone in defendants' employ", meaning that they are requiring information that a whistleblower, as an employee of the company, could gain access to.

22

ARTICLES REFERRING TO NATHAN V. TAKEDA

There have been a lot of articles written about my case but unfortunately, all of the articles were about the legal issue and nothing about the health risk. Lawyers are concerned about the "Level of Specificity Required Under Rule 9(b) in False Claims Act Whistleblower Suits" but not about the suit itself. I have seen articles from both sides, for and against; on how they feel the United States Supreme Court should rule on my case to clear up the issue. It seemed like everyone but the Solicitor General of the United States wanted the case decided but in my opinion he was concerned with the conservative leaning of the Supreme Court in 2014.

The Honorable Justice Antonin Scalia was on the Supreme Court at the time, before his death on February 13, 2016. He was thought to be one of the most conservative justices in modern times but as Stephen M. Kohn points out, "In 1999–2000, when the U.S. Chamber of Commerce and its government-contractor allies raised a Supreme Court challenge to the constitutionality of the False Claims Act (the most effective whistleblower law in the United States), Supreme Court Justice Antonin Scalia rebuked their attack, extensively citing the actions of the First Congress.

He pointed out that on July 31, 1789, our Founding Fathers enacted the first of eighteen *qui tam* laws mandating that whistle-blowers (informants) whose original information resulted in a successful enforcement action be entitled to a percentage of the collected proceeds. This is the precise model used in the False Claims Act and the other very successful whistleblower reward laws today."[1]

I KNOW I have said it before, but my case didn't get past the Motion to Dismiss phase. We never got our chance to go to trial and prove our facts of the case. Since the dosage data wasn't broken down by 30mg and 60mg until after the case began, I wasn't permitted to use it.

IN AN ARTICLE BY BRIANNA BLOODGOOD, "Particularity Discovery In *Qui Tam* Actions: A Middle Ground Approach To Pleading Fraud In The Health Care Sector" in the *University of Pennsylvania Law Review*,[2] she states:

"The circuits are divided as to what constitutes a sufficiently particular complaint in the FCA context. One approach requires that the plaintiff's complaint identify at least one false claim by time, place, content of the action, and names of actors. Defendants favor this "representative sample" approach because it places the onus on the private citizen relator to present specific factual details of the alleged fraudulent activity. This is often a heavy burden for a relator who, absent ordinary civil discovery, lacks the investigative resources of the government.

Under this standard, private plaintiffs may face difficulties pleading a representative sample of facts in a way that ensures the claim is not conclusory—in other words, that it does not require the court to make any logical leaps from the facts to find that the claim for fraud is plausible. For example, in *United States ex rel. Nathan v. Takeda Pharmaceuticals*, the complaint alleged that ninety-eight non-reimbursable prescriptions for sixty milligrams of a drug called Kapidex (samples of which Takeda provided to doctors) were submitted to the Centers for Medicare & Medicaid Services for reimbursement. The sixty milligram dose for Kapidex is not eligible for federal reimbursement for certain uses that are off-label. The relator, a sales manager for Takeda, also alleged two additional facts: the names of sixteen doctors who wrote prescriptions for Kapidex (at unknown dosages) and submitted them for reimbursement, and the fact that ninety-three percent of all prescriptions for Kapidex are for a sixty milligram dose. Nonetheless, the court dismissed the claim on Takeda's Rule 12(b)(6) motion. Allowing the case to proceed would have required the court to speculate that the specific Kapidex prescriptions of the sixteen identified doctors were in fact for sixty milligrams; such a logical leap indicated a lack of plausibility. The Takeda case illustrates that even a relator with specific information suggesting a strong possibility of fraud will struggle under the strict representative sample pleading standard given the interrelationship among Rule 8(a), Rule 9(b), and the Twombly–Iqbal plausibility standard.

The government's *amicus curiae* brief in Takeda asserted that a "strong inference" approach to pleading an FCA violation is preferable to a heightened requirement, and, in 2014, the Third Circuit joined several other circuits in adopting that more relaxed pleading standard. In courts that have adopted this approach, a plaintiff can survive a motion to dismiss by pleading facts that support a strong inference that the defendant violated the FCA. A general description of the alleged fraudulent scheme combined with such reliable indicia of fraudulent activity will suffice."[3]

AN ARTICLE WRITTEN by the American Health Lawyers Association in 2015,[4] shows the Solicitor General's brief from my case has been persuasive to courts who are being asked whether Rule 9(b) requires *qui tam* relators to plead specific examples of allegedly false claims.

"For example, in June of this year, the D.C. Circuit rejected a defense argument that Rule 9(b) requires a relator to plead "representative examples" of the false claims. In doing so, the court (quoting language from the Solicitor General's briefing in Takeda) stated that "[t]he federal government itself already has records of those payments and thus 'rarely if ever needs a relator's assistance to identify claims for payment that have been submitted [.]'" United States ex rel. Heath v. AT & T, Inc., No. 14-7094, 2015 WL 3852180, at *11 (D.C. Cir. June 23, 2015) (citation omitted). The bottom is line is that the proper application of Rule 9(b) continues to be hard-fought by litigants, and the Supreme Court will be called on again to resolve this question."[5]

THIS BRINGS up another frustrating issue, the federal government had records of what they paid for, and it would show that they paid for 60mg capsules of Dexilant! My case didn't involve private insurance companies, although this book is meant to alert all patients of the health concern in taking double the dose without ever trying the 30mg dose. The 30mg and 60mg doses were priced the same which was one of Takeda's defenses during the proceedings, but the issue is they wanted the 60mg to make sure it worked. If the patient took the 30mg dose and they still had heartburn they might get switched to another proton pump inhibitor instead of refilling their Dexilant.

IN AN ARTICLE by George Breen et al, "Supreme Court Declines to Opine on Circuit Split Over Rule 9(b) Pleading Requirements for FCA Claims",[6] they state:

"The Supreme Court's inaction leaves intact the circuit split on applying Rule 9(b) to FCA claims, as well as the attendant uncertainty among health care providers, life science companies, and any others litigating FCA actions. Because circuit courts of appeal embrace different standards for applying Rule 9(b), it is critical that litigants pursuing or defending FCA actions remain mindful of the applicable jurisdiction's approach—as circuit choice may have a dispositive difference at the motion-to-dismiss stage. Moreover, because the Fourth Circuit's Nathan decision deepens the circuit split on applying Rule 9(b) to FCA claims, litigants may find it easier to establish grounds for interlocutory appeal under 28 U.S.C. § 1292(b).

Litigants pursuing or defending *qui tam* actions must remain attuned to the significant differences in pleading requirements among circuits relative to the Rule 9(b) "particularity" requirement. Nathan clarifies the Fourth Circuit's position as aligned with the other circuits requiring FCA relators, as part of Rule 9(b), to meet a more stringent pleading standard and identify a specific false claim that was submitted for payment to a federal health care program (the Sixth, Eighth, and Eleventh Circuit approach). When litigating in circuits applying the more stringent Rule 9(b) standard, defendants should carefully consider moving to dismiss a *qui tam* complaint that fails to identify at least one specific false claim being submitted for federal health care program payment.

Nathan expands the circuit split in applying Rule 9(b) to FCA complaints. Relators alleging FCA violations in the Fourth, Sixth, Eighth, and Eleventh Circuits generally have to clear a more difficult evidentiary hurdle at the pleading stage than relators in the First, Fifth, Seventh, and Ninth Circuits. Relators in the former category may have more difficulty surviving a motion to dismiss, as they are generally required to identify a specific false claim that was submitted for federal health care program payment—a demanding standard when a whistleblower notices fraud but lacks access to submitted claims. And relators in the latter category need not produce a specific request for payment but can generally survive a motion to dismiss by alleging the details of the fraudulent scheme, bolstered by facts leading to a "strong inference" that false claims were submitted.

Because the Supreme Court denied Nathan's petition for certiorari, this split will remain in place until further Congressional or judicial action. In the interim, precedent from the Fourth Circuit, and from other circuits applying the more stringent pleading standard, continues to support the use of Rule 9(b) as a powerful gatekeeping tool."[7]

IN AN ARTICLE BY JOSEPH R. Berger, "Petitions to Supreme Court Shine Light on FCA Circuit Rulings, Fourth Circuit Case Law,"[8] which was written before the Supreme Court decided on my case, he opines:

"Implications of Nathan Petition. If the Supreme Court were to take the case and reverse the Fourth Circuit, then in the Fourth and other circuits that currently adhere strictly to Rule 9(b), a greater number of complaints could proceed past the pleading stage without the requirement to allege a particular false claim, or to plead the alleged fraud with particularity as required by the Fourth Circuit. In that event, in the Fourth Circuit, relators might take advantage of the combined effect of a loosened pleading standard and, under the Carter decision, the suspension of the statute of limitations and diminished first-to-file bar. This could make it easier for relators to resurrect stale or failed allegations and evade the FCA statute of limitations without even the need to identify a false claim at the pleading stage, imposing additional new challenges for government contractors and opening up another new floodgate for FCA lawsuits against them.

If the Supreme Court denies the petition, then the Fourth Circuit and other circuits can preserve the significant gatekeeping mechanism of Rule 9(b) at the pleading stage. If the Court takes the case and affirms the decision, then a uniformity of pleading standards could be established that preserves the Fourth Circuit's application of Rule 9(b) in FCA cases."[9]

IN AN ARTICLE by Karin Lee titled,"Linking Rule 9(b) and the FCA's First-to-File Rule to Advance the Goals Of The False Claims Act"[10] she states:

"The Fourth and Eighth Circuits' Inflexibility.—The Fourth and Eighth Circuits have shown the least flexibility in their interpretations of Rule 9(b). The Eighth Circuit applies the same restrictive 9(b) standard to both subsection (a)(1) and subsection (a)(2) claims, effectively requiring a *qui tam* relator to plead details of specific fraudulent claims that were made. Similarly, the Fourth Circuit has distanced itself from the more permissive standards. It requires details of specific claims where alleged behavior "could have led, but need not necessarily have led" to actually submitted false claims."[11]

AN ARTICLE by Michael Lockman from *The University of Chicago Law Review*, "In Defense of a Strict Pleading Standard for False Claims Act Whistleblowers",[12] he provides his opinion that while there exists a circuit split, some circuits are moving towards a loose interpretation while some are just inconsistent:

"The Erosion of the Circuit Split

Over the course of the past ten years, the circuit split has eroded in favor of the relaxed standard. Furthermore, the courts that have adhered to the strict standard have applied it inconsistently. For example, the Eighth Circuit recently abandoned its adherence to the strict standard by noting that relators who can "plead details about the defendant's billing practices and plead personal knowledge of the defendant's submission of false claims" may be excused from the strict standard. Likewise while the Sixth Circuit has not yet departed from the strict standard,'" it has indicated that the pleading standard may be relaxed "when the relator has personal knowledge that the claims were submitted by Defendants... for payment." The pleading standard as applied by the Sixth and Eighth Circuits can thus be understood as a means of distinguishing between insider and outsider relators. Approximately 25 percent of relators are outsiders such as competitors, partners, subcontractors, or outside investigators. Courts may not perceive such outsider relators as those for whom the *qui tam* provisions were originally enacted. The Third and Tenth Circuits have also abandoned the strict standard. Likewise, the Eleventh Circuit, once a bastion of the strict standard, recently tempered its pleading rule, noting that "alternative means are also available to satisfy [Rule 9(b)]." The pleading standard remains an open question in the Seventh Circuit, and despite Seventh Circuit precedent suggesting adherence to the relaxed standard, "district courts in the Seventh Circuit have applied both competing interpretations."

Some circuits have carved out their own middle grounds. The Fourth Circuit recently held that if the "defendant's actions, as alleged and as reasonably inferred from the allegations, could have led, but need not necessarily have led, to the submission of false claims, a relator must allege with particularity that specific false claims actually were presented to the government for payment." In other words, unless the relator can plead particularized firsthand knowledge of an "integrated scheme in which presentment of a claim for payment was a necessary result," a complaint lacking specific examples of allegedly false claims will fail to meet the Rule 9(b) threshold.

The First Circuit's nuanced relaxed standard also bears mentioning. This pleading standard distinguishes between allegations that a defendant filed false claims and allegations that a defendant induced third parties to file false claims. With regard to the latter, a relator may satisfy Rule 9(b) by providing factual or

statistical evidence but need not necessarily provide particularized details concerning each false claim. "[13]

AN ARTICLE by Vann Bentley from *The Georgetown Law Review*,
"Getting Particular: Finding the Appropriate False Claims Act
Pleading Standard Post-Nathan v. Takeda Pharmaceuticals"[14]
states:

"Because the differing Rule 9(b) pleading standards adopted
by the circuits can determine the fate of an FCA complaint, it is
imperative for the Supreme Court to clarify the issue. Recently,
the relator in Nathan appealed his case to the Supreme Court,
but the Court denied certiorari. However, before declining to
take the case, the Court asked Solicitor General Donald Verrilli
to submit a brief on behalf of the federal government. The Solicitor General's position was that Nathan was not the appropriate
case for the Supreme Court to use as a vehicle to clarify the Rule
9(b) issue because it is unclear whether the relator in Nathan
would have been able to satisfy 9(b) even with the more lenient
standard, and the Court should take up the issue in a case where
the pleading standard is more clearly outcome determinative.
This brief presumably helped the Court decide not to take the
case. However, the Solicitor General's brief did make clear that
the position of the United States was that Rule 9(b) should not
be held to an overly rigid standard. Perhaps, this is not a
surprising position for the government to take, given that it has
an interest in being able to aggressively sue parties who it
believes have committed fraud against it. However, the brief does
bring up some useful arguments for rejecting a rigid interpretation of 9(b).

The Court should take up this issue and adopt a more lenient
reading of Rule 9(b) for several reasons: (1) An overly strict
reading of Rule 9(b) would make it very difficult for legitimate
FCA *qui tam* suits to survive; (2) a strict interpretation is inconsis-

tent with the text of the FCA; and (3), a strict interpretation is inconsistent with the purposes of Rule 9(b).

As the Solicitor General notes in his brief, an overly restrictive Rule 9(b) standard would "hinder the ability of *qui tam* relators to perform the role that Congress intended them to play in detection and remediation of fraud against the United States." The brief gives the example of an employee who wants to blow the whistle on his employer's fraudulent practices. The employee may have enough information to know that his employer is engaged in fraud in their dealings with the government, but may not be privy to the employer's billing practices. Under the standard adopted in Nathan, it seems likely that this employee's complaint would be doomed, even if his information outside of the billing process was quite useful. The Solicitor General makes the interesting point that requiring relators to know which specific claims were filed to the government may not even be useful, as the government usually already has that information available to it. Having one step in the fraudulent process (the actual billing to the government) be dispositive over any other information the relator may possess seems arbitrary and will prevent some merited FCA claims from succeeding, which will undermine the goal of the FCA to rectify fraud against the government.

An overly strict 9(b) standard also seems to contradict the text of the FCA. The Third Circuit in Foglia noted that the strict interpretation of Rule 9(b) favored by the Fourth, Sixth, Eighth, and Eleventh Circuits is inconsistent with the text of the FCA, which does not require that the exact content of the false claims in question be shown. Therefore, the Court says, to hold relators to this standard at the pleading stage would require them to present documentation that they are not even required to present at trial. Once again, having the actual presentment of claims to the government serve as the one piece of evidence that is unavoidable seems like an arbitrary decision by the courts. While the statute does seek to make only those liable who have presented these false claims, there are other pieces of evidence that can lead to this same result. Evidence of a fraudulent scheme to defraud the government that reasonably led to these claims (as in the more lenient 9(b) standard of the First, Third, Fifth, and Ninth Circuits) would seem to accomplish this same goal and not violate the text of the FCA. Therefore, relators should not be arbitrarily limited by a requirement for one specific type of evidence that is not present in the text of the FCA.

Finally, the courts who have adopted the strict interpretation of Rule 9(b) seem to ignore the purposes of Rule 9(b). The four important purposes of the "pleading with particularity" requirement as laid out in Nathan, are to protect against frivolous lawsuits, to protect defendant from suits in which all the facts are learned in discovery, to give the defendant notice of his alleged wrongdoings, and to protect the defendant from reputational harm. But all of these purposes seem to still be served under the nuanced Rule 9(b) interpretation of the First, Third, Fifth, Seventh, and Ninth Circuits. Those circuits do not relax the requirement that the relator plead facts with particularity; they just do not specify as strictly which facts the relator must plead with particularity. The standard set in those circuits still requires facts to be pled with particularity that demonstrate that false claims were likely submitted to the government. A relator is not going to be able to pass this standard with a frivolous lawsuit or a lawsuit devoid of any facts at the pleading stage. Furthermore, for a fraudulent scheme to meet the 9(b) standard even in these more lenient circuits, the relator still must allege enough facts to give the defendant notice of his wrongdoings. If frivolous lawsuits are not allowed, then the concern about reputational harm of the defendant is also not implicated here. Because the purposes of Rule 9(b) do not require the stricter standard set by the Fourth, Sixth, Eighth, and Eleventh Circuits, the Supreme Court should reject this interpretation."[15]

. . .

AN ARTICLE by Cameron S. Hamrick, "Third Circuit Adds to Circuit Split on Rule 9(b)'s Particularity Requirement in the Context of an FCA Claim"[16], mentions not only the Circuit split but how the Solicitor General's brief is influencing the divide.

"The Third Circuit did not engage in a lengthy analysis of the two approaches. Instead, the court cited one of its previous decisions in which it noted that it had never held that a plaintiff must identify a specific claim for payment at the pleading stage to state a claim for relief. In addition, the court cited DOJ's amicus brief regarding the certiorari petition in Takeda Pharmaceuticals, which argued that the "rigid" pleading standard required by the Fourth, Sixth, Eighth, and Eleventh Circuits is "unsupported by Rule 9(b) and undermines the FCA's effectiveness as a tool to combat fraud against the United States." The Third Circuit concluded that "[i]n so far as the purpose of Rule 9(b) is to 'provide defendants with fair notice of plaintiffs' claims,'" the approach followed by the "First, Fifth, and Eleventh Circuits will suffice."

Turning to the relator's allegations, the Court noted that "[t]his is a close case as to meeting the requirements of Rule 9(b)," but held that the relator had provided sufficient facts to meet those requirements. The Court stated that its conclusion was supported by the fact that only the defendant has access to the documents that could "easily prove the claim one way or another.""[17]

23

LUPRON

L upron was promoted by TAP Pharmaceuticals and eventually became part of Abbott Labs portfolio of drugs when TAP was dissolved in 2008.

Lupron was approved by the FDA in 1985. That same year TAP Pharmaceuticals began promotion of Lupron as a daily subcutaneous injection for prostate cancer and infertility which could be self-administered by the patient. According to Dr. Gerald Weisberg, Lupron sales were minimal.[1] Takeda research developed Lupron Depot in 1989 which is a once a month formulation of Lupron that needed to be administered in a physician's office through an injection. By providing the injection in the office, the physician can bill for the procedure on top of the charge for the medicine.

In her book, "An American Sickness: How Healthcare Became Big Business and How You Can Take It Back"[2], Elisabeth Rosenthal states that when other companies brought cheaper drugs to the market, TAP came up with a program to provide free samples that the physicians could administer and still bill for. Rosenthal explains that TAP sent physicians promotional material, specifically one called "the Lupron checkbook" to show how much money they could earn by prescribing and injecting Lupron. Ms. Rosenthal also presented that the president of the American Urological Association made his organization aware that charging for free samples could be illegal.

Dr. Gerald Weisberg is an Endocrinologist by trade and was the Head of Clinical Research for Lupron at TAP Pharmaceuticals from 1992 to 1996. Dr. Weisberg brought up his concern about encouraging physicians to bill for free samples and was then labeled a "disgruntled employee" and fired. In an ABC News article[3], Dr. Weisberg stated, "We are talking about schemes quite possible developed at the TAP home office, clearly implemented through the efforts of people in the TAP home office and then given to people out in the field."

Doug Durand was Vice-President of Sales at TAP Pharmaceuticals at the time and became a whistleblower to stop the scheme. TAP settled with the government for over $875 million and agreed to a Corporate Integrity Agreement intended to keep the company clean.

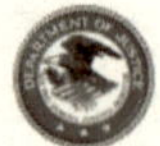

FOR IMMEDIATE RELEASE

CIV

WEDNESDAY, OCTOBER 3, 2001

(202) 514-2007

WWW.USDOJ.GOV

TDD (202) 514-1888

TAP PHARMACEUTICAL PRODUCTS INC.

AND SEVEN OTHERS CHARGED WITH HEALTH CARE CRIMES; COMPANY AGREES TO PAY $875 MILLION TO SETTLE CHARGES

Boston, MA... United States Attorney Michael J. Sullivan, Department of Health and Human Services Inspector General Janet Rehnquist, Assistant Inspector General for Investigations and Director of the Department of Defense Criminal Investigation Service Carol Levy, and Special Agent in Charge of the Federal Bureau of Investigation in New England Charles S. Prouty, announced today that:

(1) **TAP Pharmaceutical Products Inc.** ("TAP"), a major American pharmaceutical manufacturer, has agreed to pay $875,000,000 to resolve criminal charges and civil liabilities in connection with its fraudulent drug pricing and marketing conduct with regard to Lupron, a drug sold by **TAP** primarily for treatment of advanced prostate cancer in men. The global agreement includes:

(a) **TAP** has agreed to plead guilty to a conspiracy to violate the PrescriptionDrug Marketing Act and to pay a $290,000,000 criminal fine, the largest criminal fine ever in a health care fraud prosecution. The plea agreement between the United States and **TAP** specifically states that **TAP**'s criminal conduct caused losses of $145,000,000.

(b) **TAP** has agreed to settle its federal civil False Claims Act liabilities and to pay the U.S. Government $559,483,560 for filing false and fraudulent claims with the Medicare and Medicaid programs as a result of **TAP**'s fraudulent drug pricing schemes and sales and marketing misconduct.

(c) **TAP** has agreed to settle its civil liabilities to the fifty states and the District of Columbia and to pay them $25,516,440 for filing false and fraudulent claims with the states, as a result of **TAP**'s drug pricing and marketing misconduct, and from **TAP**'s failure to provide the state Medicaid programs **TAP**'s best price for those drugs as required by law.

(d) **TAP** has agreed to comply with the terms of a sweeping corporate integrity agreement which, among other things, significantly changes the manner in which **TAP** supervises its marketing and sales staff, and ensures that **TAP** will report to the Medicare and Medicaid programs the true average sale price for drugs reimbursed by those programs.

(2) A federal grand jury returned an indictment unsealed today, charging one physician and six **TAP** managers with conspiracy to pay kickbacks to doctors and other customers, conspiracy to defraud the state Medicaid programs on **TAP**'s obligation to sell products to those programs at its best price, and conspiracy to

violate the Prescription Drug Marketing Act by causing free samples to be illegally billed to the Medicare program. The indictment charges that the **TAP** defendants offered to give things of value, including free drugs, so-called educational grants, trips to resorts, free consulting services, medical equipment, and forgiveness of debt, to physicians and other customers to obtain their referrals of prescriptions for Lupron to Medicare program beneficiaries, in violation of the anti-kickback statute. The indictment also charges that the **TAP** defendants aided and abetted, and caused the billings to hundreds of elderly Medicare program beneficiaries and to the Medicare program directly, for thousands of free samples of Lupron, used in the treatment of prostate cancer, in violation of the Prescription Drug Marketing Act.

The seven individuals charged in the indictment unsealed today are:

(1) **ALAN MACKENZIE**, age 49, of 27068 Wellington Court, Barrington, Illinois, and formerly Vice President of Sales for **TAP**.

(2) **JANICE SWIRSKI**, age 40, of 6 Bellingham Drive, Chestnut Hill, Massachusetts, and formerly a National Account Manager with **TAP**.

(3) **HENRY VAN MOURICK**, age 43, of 23 Golfwood Court, Roseville, California, and currently a District Manager employed by **TAP**.

(4) **DONNA TOM**, age 37, of 141 East 56th Street, New York, New York, and formerly a District Manager employed by **TAP**.

(5) **KIMBERLEE CHASE**, age 35, of 108 Dedham Street, Dover, Massachusetts, and formerly a District Manager employed by **TAP**.

(6) **DAVID GUIDO**, age 30, of 131 New London Road, Colchester, Connecticut, and currently a Hospital Account Executive employed by **TAP**.

(7) **DR. JOHN ROMANO**, age 48, of 110 Long Pond Road, Plymouth, Massachusetts, an urologist with a practice in Plymouth, Massachusetts.

Prior to yesterday's indictment, four other physicians have been charged and have pleaded guilty in this investigation: Dr. Rodney Mannion, a urologist practicing in LaPorte and Michigan City, Indiana, was charged on February 28, 2000 with healthcare fraud. Dr. Mannion pleaded guilty to that charge on April 25, 2000. Dr. Jacob Zamstein, a urologist practicing in Bloomfield, Connecticut, was charged on November 3, 2000 with healthcare fraud and pleaded guilty on December 27, 2000. Dr. Joseph Spinella, a urologist practicing in Bristol, Connecticut, was charged on December 8, 2000 with healthcare fraud and pleaded guilty on March 29, 2001. Dr. Joel Olstein, a urologist practicing in Lewiston, Maine, was charged on April 11, 2001 with healthcare fraud and pleaded guilty on July 18, 2001.

Lupron is marketed by **TAP** primarily for the treatment of prostate cancer. Lupron is identical in effectiveness to the drug Zolodex, produced by a competitor, which was also available for prescription in the 1990s. While Medicare does not pay for most drugs needed by Medicare beneficiaries, Medicare does cover drugs, such as Lupron, that must be injected under the supervision of a physician. Medicare paid for 80% of either the urologist's charge for Lupron or the average wholesale price reported by **TAP**, whichever was lower, and the patient was responsible for the remaining 20% as a copayment.

As part of its civil allegations, the Government alleged that throughout the1990s, **TAP** set and controlled the price at which the Medicare program reimbursed physicians for the prescription of Lupron by reporting its average wholesale price ("AWP"). The AWP reported by TAP was significantly higher than the average sales price **TAP** offered physicians and other customers for the drug. The Government alleged that **TAP** marketed the spread between its discounted prices paid by physicians and the significantly higher Medicare reimbursement based on AWP as an inducement to physicians to obtain their Lupron business. The Government further alleged that **TAP** concealed the true discounted prices paid by physicians from Medicare, and falsely advised physicians to report the higher AWP rather than their real discounted price for the drug. The Government further alleged that **TAP** set its AWPs of Lupron at levels far higher than the price for which wholesalers or distributors actually sold the drug, resulting in falsely inflated prices that were neither the physician's actual cost nor the true wholesaler's average price.

"The Medicare and Medicaid drug programs are bulwarks against the financial hardship that can be caused by the need for life-saving medical treatments," said Robert D. McCallum, Jr., Assistant Attorney General for the Justice Department's Civil Division. "These programs cannot afford abuses that enrich doctors or drug companies at the expense of taxpayers and patients. This settlement agreement and the compliance steps that TAP has agreed to take will reinforce the government's long-standing objective of paying Medicare and Medicaid providers for the reasonable costs of the drugs they administer."

"The urologists and the TAP employees who knowingly participated in this broad conspiracy took advantage of older Americans suffering from prostate cancer. The indictment unsealed today alleges that TAP employees sought to influence the doctors' decisions about what drug to prescribe to patients by giving them kickbacks and bribes, from free samples to free consulting services to expensive trips to golf and ski resorts to so-called educational grants," said U.S. Attorney Sullivan. "In all instances where the kickbacks worked to ensure the prescription of TAP's product Lupron, the Medicare Program and the elderly Americans suffering from prostate cancer paid more for their care than if the doctor had prescribed the competitor's product."

"Medicare beneficiaries and all American patients need to get the right pharmaceuticals, based on medical criteria, and at a fair price. This is crucial both to ensure good quality health care and to use our resources effectively. Today's settlement is a clear message that the federal government will protect the best interests of beneficiaries and taxpayers," said HHS Secretary Tommy G. Thompson.

"This prosecution has resulted in the largest criminal and civil recoveries in any health care fraud case in the country. The fraud schemes used by TAP Pharmaceuticals and others impacts significantly on the integrity of TRICARE, the Department of Defense's healthcare system," stated DCIS Special Agent in Charge Edward Bradley. "Healthcare fraud increases patients' costs and negatively effects the delivery of health care services to over 8 million military members, retirees, and their dependents."

The indictment unsealed today against the seven individuals alleges that inducements to physicians included free products; free consulting services; trips to expensive golf and ski resorts; money disguised as "educational grants," but in fact was used and intended to be used for many purposes, including cocktail party bar tabs, office Christmas parties, medical equipment, travel expenses for urologists and their staff to attend conferences; and discounts on Lupron sold to treat endometriosis in women to effect a lower price on Lupron used in the treatment of men with prostate cancer.

The investigation commenced in the District of Massachusetts in 1997 after a urologist employed by Tufts Associated Health Maintenance Organization ("Tufts HMO") in Waltham, Dr. Joseph Gerstein, reported to law enforcement authorities that he had been offered an educational grant if he would reverse a decision he had made on behalf of Tufts that it would only cover the less expensive drug Zoladex. As charged in the indictment, **SWIRSKI** and **CHASE** met with Dr. Gerstein after he began working with the FBI and the Office of Inspector General, and during those meetings, offered him $65,000 in educational grants that he could use for any purpose "whatever," together with discounts on other products, if he would reverse Tufts' decision not to include Lupron on its formulary for treating patients that it insured who were suffering from prostate cancer. The investigation was also triggered by a civil False Claims Act suit filed in 1996 by Douglas Durand, after he had quit his employment at TAP as Vice President of Sales, after just one year because of his concerns about the illegal marketing conduct of some of **TAP**'s employees.

The civil False Claims Act provides that where persons submit, cause others to submit, or conspire to submit, false or fraudulent claims to the United States

Government, including its federal health care programs, the Government is entitled to recover treble damages and $5,500 to $11,000 for each false or fraudulent claim submitted. Private individuals, like Dr. Gerstein and Douglas Durand, are allowed to file whistleblower suits under the False Claims Act to bring the government information about wrongdoing, and if the government is successful in resolving or litigating their claims, to share in the recovery by receiving generally 15% to 25% of the amount recovered. As a part of today's resolution, those two individuals together with Tufts Associated HMO will share as whistleblowers, pursuant to the Congressional directive in the False Claims Act, 17% of the civil recovery, or an amount of approximately $95 million.

"The payment by TAP of nearly $900 million including the highest criminal fine ever imposed on any health care company, and the indictment of the six TAP employees sends a very strong signal to the pharmaceutical industry that it best police its employees' conduct and deal strongly with those who would gain sales at the expense of the health care programs for the poor and the elderly and the persons insured by those programs," said U.S. Attorney Sullivan.

As part of a condition for doing business in the future with providers who are members of the Medicare and Medicaid programs, **TAP** agreed to enter into an extensive Corporate Integrity Agreement. That agreement provides for significant training of **TAP**'s sales and marketing employees and changes in supervision and controls. It also requires **TAP** to report to the Medicare and Medicaid programs accurate pricing information showing **TAP**'s true average sales price.

"In recent years, the pharmaceutical industry has come under increasing scrutiny for its pricing, sales, and marketing practices. The OIG, together with other government agencies, will use all available enforcement authorities, where appropriate, to address these practices," said HHS Inspector General Janet Rehnquist.

The entire amount of the $290 million criminal fine paid by TAP will go to the Department of Justice's Crime Victims Fund. The Fund was established in 1984 by the Victims of Crime Act ("VOCA") and serves as a major funding source for victim services throughout the country. Each year, millions of dollars are deposited into this fund from criminal fines, forfeited bail bonds, penalty fees, and special assessments collected by U.S. Attorney's Offices, U.S. Courts, and the Bureau of Prisons. State assistance programs use VOCA funds to provide or contract for services to victims of rape, drunk driving, child abuse, domestic violence, homicide, and other crimes. Victims of federal, as well as state crimes, are eligible to receive VOCA-funded services.

The investigation is continuing.

The investigation has been conducted by the agents from the Federal Bureau of Investigation, the Office of Investigations for the Office of Inspector General for the Department of Health and Human Services, the Food and Drug Administration's Office of Criminal Investigations and the Department of Defense's Defense Criminal Investigation Service. On the criminal side, the investigation and prosecution are being handled by Assistant U.S. Attorney Michael K. Loucks, Health Care Fraud Chief. On the civil side, the investigation and prosecution are being handled by Assistant U.S. Attorney Susan Winkler, assisted by Department of Justice Trial Attorney T. Reed Stephens. The Corporate Integrity Agreement was negotiated by Office of General Counsel, Office of Inspector General Assistant Counsel Mary Riordan.

Press Contact: Samantha Martin, (617) 748-3139

###

01-513

24

ACTOS (PIOGLITAZONE)

Actos (pioglitazone) is an oral type 2 diabetes medication that helps control blood sugar levels. Actos was approved in the U.S. in 1999 in the drug class called Thiazolidinediones (TZD).

In 2015, Takeda Pharmaceuticals agreed to one of the largest pharmaceutical settlements in U.S. history. Takeda paid $2.4 billion to settle 9,000 lawsuits for life-threatening injuries including bladder cancer and heart failure, while not admitting any guilt and standing by the effectiveness of Actos. There are still lawsuits that refused to settle and are on-going.

In 2014, a jury in Louisiana awarded Terrence Allen $9 billion in punitive damages and $1.5 million in compensatory damages for his bladder cancer that was caused by taking Actos. Even though a judge later reduced the total award down to $36.8 million, the verdict sent a strong signal to Takeda.

The judge in the above *Allen v. Takeda* trial[1] was the U.S. District Judge Rebecca Doherty. Judge Doherty said that Takeda intentionally destroyed evidence that would have helped the defense. She stated, "There is no dispute in this case as to the intentional nature of the defendants' document destruction."

"The absence of those files can be reasonably assumed to have prejudiced Mr. and Mrs. Allen from presenting a full and complete picture of Takeda's actions and will prejudice the [plaintiffs steering committee] within this MDL, as those documents are forever lost, and the electronically generated or stored information was deleted and cannot be fully reconstituted."

THE MAJORITY of Actos lawsuits state Takeda knew about the concern of bladder cancer but did not warn the public. The FDA did not make Takeda remove Actos from the market but required Takeda to update the Actos product information to include the potential of an increased risk of bladder cancer.

THE U.S. FDA issued a safety warning:[2]

Safety Announcement.

[6-15-2011] The U.S. Food and Drug Administration (FDA) is informing the public that use of the diabetes medication Actos (pioglitazone) for more than one year may be associated with an increased risk of bladder cancer. Information about this risk will be added to the Warnings and Precautions section of the label for pioglitazone-containing medicines. The patient Medication Guide for these medicines will also be revised to include information on the risk of bladder cancer.

Facts about pioglitazone

• Sold as a single-ingredient product under the brand name Actos. Also sold in combination with metformin (Actoplus Met, Actoplus Met XR) and glimepiride (Duetact).

• Used along with diet bond exercise to improve control of blood sugar in adults with type 2 diabetes mellitus.

• From January 2010 through October 2010, approximately 2.3 million patients filled a prescription for a pioglitazone-containing product from outpatient retail pharmacies.[2]

This safety information is based on FDA's review of data from a planned five-year interim analysis of an ongoing, ten-year epidemiological study1, described in FDA's September 2010 ongoing safety review and in the Data Summary below. The five-year results showed that although there was no overall increased risk of bladder cancer with pioglitazone use, an increased risk of bladder cancer was noted among patients with the longest exposure to pioglitazone, and in those exposed to the highest cumulative dose of pioglitazone.

FDA is also aware of a recent epidemiological study conducted in France which suggests an increased risk of bladder cancer with pioglitazone. Based on the results of this study, France has suspended the use of pioglitazone and Germany has recommended not to start pioglitazone in new patients.

FDA recommends that healthcare professionals should:

•Not use pioglitazone in patients with active bladder cancer.

•Use pioglitazone with caution in patients with a prior history of bladder cancer. The benefits of blood sugar control with pioglitazone should be weighed against the unknown risks for cancer recurrence.

FDA will continue to evaluate data from the ongoing ten-year epidemiological study. The Agency will also conduct a comprehensive review of the results from the French study. FDA will update the public when more information becomes available.

THE ACTOS TRIALS and settlement negotiation was happening during the same time as my whistleblower case. Having to listen to Takeda and their lawyers talk about how patient safety is their number one priority, all while they are still promoting Dexilant at double the dose troubled me. I wanted to scream at the top of my lungs about what is going on, but I knew I had to remain quiet. Takeda was caught destroying documents that could have included incriminating evidence on their knowledge about bladder cancer, and they claim patient safety is their number one priority. If patient safety is their number one priority why are they promoting Dexilant at the double the dose while having a safety warning to use the lowest dose for the shortest duration of time?

To build employee loyalty they came up with what they call, Takeda-ism. Takeda promotes their Takeda-ism as Patient – Trust – Reputation – Business. Words are cheap.

25

CONCLUSION - CALL TO ACTION

Whether you are a patient that has been on Dexilant, a physician that has been called on by a Dexilant sales representative, or just a concerned citizen, my ask of you is to contact your elected representatives and demand an update to the False Claims Act. It has been done before.

As recently as 2009, the United States Congress added an amendment to the False Claims Act. On May 20, 2009 the Fraud Enforcement and Recovery Act (FERA) was signed into law by President Obama. The FERA was in response to a U.S. Supreme Court decision in *Allison Engine Co. v. United States ex rel. Sanders.*[1]

Jeremy E. Gersh states in, "Saying What They Mean: The False Claims Act Amendments in the Wake of Allison Engine",[2] Congress did not agree with the Supreme Court's decision in Allison Engine, and passed the amendment to clarify the law which the court will interpret in the future. "FERA completely rewrote § 3729 to return the statute to Congress's original intent. First, Congress rewrote § 3729(a)(2) by removing the phrase "paid or approved by the Government," and focused on "a false or fraudulent claim." Further, Congress added a materiality requirement to the FCA, defining materiality as "having a natural tendency to influence, or be capable of influencing, the payment or receipt of money or property." Now, a false statement only needs to be "material to a false or fraudulent claim," and there is no element of intent."

THE CIRCUIT COURTS are split on how to decide the Rule 9(b) issue and until the law is resolved, good people trying to do the right thing will continue to be rejected. The False Claims Act is meant to encourage companies to be honest, by offering rewards to employees for bringing fraudulent activities to light. If whistle-blowers continue to be denied their day in court, profit could be encouraged over safety.

As we learned in elementary school, the legislative branch (Congress) writes the law and the judicial branch interprets the law. It is clear that the judicial branch is having trouble interpreting an important part of the False Claims Act, thereby requiring Congress to add another amendment.

Whistleblowers are putting themselves and their careers on the line trying to do the right thing. Often, the issue they are trying to expose is a safety concern potentially effecting thousands of people. Public safety should be a priority for our elected officials, and clarifying the FCA can have a positive impact on protecting Americans.

American's don't like to hear that a multi-billion dollar international company won a court case on, what can be called a technicality, while putting American lives at risk.

Once I have collected the data at www.appleQD.com we will have information that they can't ignore. We need to look at the big picture. Clarifying the False Claims Act isn't going to help my case, it is lost as far as the courts are concerned. My goal is to make sure the next whistleblower who is putting themselves on the line to help us, succeeds!

There are several ways to contact your elected officials;

The United States House of Representatives:
https://www.house.gov/representatives/find-your-representative

The United States Senate:
https://www.senate.gov/reference/common/faq/How_to_correspond_senators.htm

And this link can help you contact your federal, state, and local officials:
https://www.usa.gov/elected-officials

I WANT to take you back to my two goals for writing this book:

(1) to make the public aware of a potential health risk that could affect thousands of Americans, and

(2) to advocate for an amendment to the False Claims Act to enable future success in whistleblower suits.

I HOPE, in your eyes, that I have achieved my goals.

THANK YOU!

Noah

26

APPLEQD

AppleQD.com is designed to provide information based on what the average person should know about the healthcare system. **This site is for informational purposes only and NOT medical advice**

I define AppleQD as "an apple a day" using the Latin *quaque die* which translates to "one a day". QD is a normal term for a physician to write on a prescription so the pharmacist and patient know that the medication is to be taken once a day.

The phrase, "An apple a day keeps the doctor away" is something we learn as children to encourage a healthy diet and I plan to take that a step further with this site.

I have been using AppleQD for years and finally decided to trademark it and create the website.

Regarding Dexilant and bone fractures, there aren't any published studies on this data. Despite the required study by Takeda, no results have been posted by the FDA, which is curious given that the required deadline was years ago. Since the data hasn't been collected, I will be seeking independent data on my website: www.appleqd.com. It is reasonable that people experienced broken bones but have not attributed it to taking high doses of Dexilant. Using the amount of literature on high dose PPI's, along with the FDA concerns, and the millions of Dexilant prescriptions filled, it should be enough to encourage further investigation. The literature shows that bones can become brittle during long-term use of high dose PPI's. If you have experienced a broken bone while on Dexilant 60mg I would encourage you to inform your physician and also go to my website, www.appleqd.-com, to add yourself to the list. The information you should provide is:

    -Your name and contact information including email address
    -Dates you took Dexilant
    -Dosage strength of Dexilant
    -Date and bone broken

REGARDLESS IF YOU have had an adverse event, I will also have an area for you to sign a petition demanding the clarification of the False Claims Act, and the ability to sign up for a newsletter to hear updates.

THANK YOU!

Noah

NOTES

Preface

1. Author
   U.S. Facts
   Article title:
   Topic: Pharmaceutical Industry in the U.S.
   Website title:
   www.statista.com
   URL:
   https://www.statista.com/topics/1719/pharmaceutical-industry/
2. *The Journal of Clinical Endocrinology & Metabolism*, Volume 103, Issue 9, 1 September 2018, Pages 3205–3214, https://doi.org/10.1210/jc.2017-02656
3. https://www.accessdata.fda.gov/drugsatfda_docs/nda/2009/022287s000TOC.cfm
4. https://clinicaltrials.gov/ct2/show/results/NCT01216293?view=results
5. Yang Y, Lewis JD, Epstein S, Metz DC. Long-term Proton Pump Inhibitor Therapy and Risk of Hip Fracture. *JAMA*. 2006;296(24):2947–2953. doi:10.1001/jama.296.24.2947
6. Brauer CA, Coca-Perraillon M, Cutler DM, Rosen AB. Incidence and Mortality of Hip Fractures in the United States. *JAMA*. 2009;302(14):1573–1579. doi:10.1001/jama.2009.1462
7. https://www.accessdata.fda.gov/drugsatfda_docs/nda/2009/022287s000TOC.cfm
8. https://www.drugs.com/stats/dexilant

1. Proof!

1. Sonnenberg, A., & El-Serag, H. B. (1999). Clinical epidemiology and natural history of gastroesophageal reflux disease. *The Yale journal of biology and medicine*, 72(2-3), 81-92.

2. $42 BILLION

1. https://www.drugs.com/stats/dexilant

3. The Pharmaceutical Industry

1. **Article title:**
   The changing role of the pharmaceutical representative
   Website title:
   Center for Health Journalism
   URL:
   https://www.centerforhealthjournalism.org/2017/04/08/changing-role-
   pharmaceutical-representative
2. **Author**
   John Abramson
   Year published:
   2014
   Book title:
   Overdosed america
   City:
   [Place of publication not identified]
   Publisher:
   Harper Perennial
3. https://www.medreps.com/medical-sales-careers/2017-pharmaceutical-
   sales-salary-report
4. **Author**
   Elisabeth Rosenthal
   Year published:
   2017
   Book title:
   An American sickness
5. http://pharmaceuticalcommerce.com/brand-marketing-communications/
   sales-rep-count-holds-relatively-steady-70000-says-zs/
6. https://www.medreps.com/medical-sales-careers/2017-pharmaceutical-
   sales-salary-report

4. The Food and Drug Administration

1. https://www.fda.gov/drugs/developmentapprovalprocess/
   howdrugsaredevelopedandapproved/approvalapplications/
   newdrugapplicationnda/default.htm
2. https://www.accessdata.fda.gov/drugsatfda_docs/nda/
   2009/022287s000TOC.cfm
3. https://clinicaltrials.gov/ct2/show/results/NCT01216293?view=results

5. HIPAA

1. https://www.hhs.gov/hipaa/index.html

6. TAP Pharmaceuticals

1. https://www.justice.gov/archive/opa/pr/2001/October/513civ.htm
2. https://www.mayoclinic.org/diseases-conditions/heartburn/expert-answers/heartburn-gerd/faq-20057894
3. https://www.accessdata.fda.gov/drugsatfda_docs/nda/2009/022287s000TOC.cfm
4. Author
   Angela Duckworth
   Year published:
   2017
   Book title:
   Grit
   City:
   [Place of publication not identified]
   Publisher:
   Vermilion

7. Prevacid

1. https://www.sec.gov/Archives/edgar/data/1114448/000110465909032651/a09-13504_16k.htm

8. Dexilant

1. https://www.accessdata.fda.gov/drugsatfda_docs/nda/2009/022287s000TOC.cfm
2. https://www.fda.gov/safety/medwatch/howtoreport/ucm053087.htm
3. https://clinicaltrials.gov/ct2/show/results/NCT01216293?view=results
4. Sonnenberg, A., & El-Serag, H. B. (1999). Clinical epidemiology and natural history of gastroesophageal reflux disease. *The Yale journal of biology and medicine*, 72(2-3), 81-92.
5. https://onlinelibrary.wiley.com/doi/abs/10.1002/pds.1825
6. Author
   Muriel R. Gillick
   Year published:
   2009

Article title:

Controlling Off-Label Medication Use

Journal title:

Annals of Internal Medicine

Issue number:

5

Volume number:

150

Pages:

344

7. **Author**

Gardiner Harris

Article title:

New Drug Label Rule Is Intended to Reduce Medical Errors

Website title:

Nytimes.com

URL:

https://www.nytimes.com/2006/01/19/us/new-drug-label-rule-is-intended-to-reduce-medical-errors.html

8. **Article title:**

Do Doctors Read Drug Warning Labels?

Website title:

Cbsnews.com

URL:

https://www.cbsnews.com/news/do-doctors-read-drug-warning-labels/

9. https://jamanetwork.com/journals/jama/article-abstract/193366

10. Ratner, Mark, and Trisha Gura. "Off-label or off-limits? Off-label prescribing is a fundamental fact of life of healthcare systems, but the promotion of off-label uses by drug sponsors is a fundamental sin. Regulators, legislators and drug makers are wrestling to find the right balance." *Nature Biotechnology*, vol. 26, no. 8, 2008, p. 867+

11. Ratner, Mark, and Trisha Gura. "Off-label or off-limits? Off-label prescribing is a fundamental fact of life of healthcare systems, but the promotion of off-label uses by drug sponsors is a fundamental sin. Regulators, legislators and drug makers are wrestling to find the right balance." *Nature Biotechnology*, vol. 26, no. 8, 2008, p. 867+

9. Dexilant and Bone Fractures

1. https://www.fda.gov/Drugs/DrugSafety/PostmarketDrugSafetyInformationforPatientsandProviders/ucm213206.htm

2. Yang Y, Lewis JD, Epstein S, Metz DC. Long-term Proton Pump Inhibitor

Therapy and Risk of Hip Fracture. *JAMA.* 2006;296(24):2947–2953. doi:10.1001/jama.296.24.2947

3. **Author**

   Liwei Wang

   Year published:

   2017

   Article title:

   Proton Pump Inhibitors and the Risk for Fracture at Specific Sites: Data Mining of the FDA Adverse Event Reporting System

   Journal title:

   Scientific Reports

   Issue number:

   1

   Volume number:

   7

4. Yang Y, Lewis JD, Epstein S, Metz DC. Long-term Proton Pump Inhibitor Therapy and Risk of Hip Fracture. *JAMA.* 2006;296(24):2947–2953. doi:10.1001/jama.296.24.2947

5. Complications of Proton Pump Inhibitor Therapy

   Vaezi, Michael F. et al.

   Gastroenterology , Volume 153 , Issue 1 , 35 - 48

6. *The Journal of Clinical Endocrinology & Metabolism*, Volume 103, Issue 9, 1 September 2018, Pages 3205–3214, https://doi.org/10.1210/jc.2017-02656

7. **Author**

   S. D. Martinez

   Year published:

   2003

   Article title:

   Non-erosive reflux disease (NERD) - acid reflux and symptom patterns

   Journal title:

   Alimentary Pharmacology and Therapeutics

   Issue number:

   4

   Volume number:

   17

   Pages:

   537-545

8. https://www.accessdata.fda.gov/drugsatfda_docs/nda/2009/022287s000TOC.cfm

9. https://www.accessdata.fda.gov/drugsatfda_docs/nda/2009/022287s000TOC.cfm

10. https://www.accessdata.fda.gov/drugsatfda_docs/nda/2009/022287s000TOC.cfm

11. https://www.accessdata.fda.gov/drugsatfda_docs/nda/
2009/022287s000TOC.cfm
12. https://clinicaltrials.gov/ct2/show/results/NCT01216293

10. Tatum v. Takeda Pharmaceuticals

1. https://www.drugwatch.com/proton-pump-inhibitors/lawsuits/
2. https://scholar.google.com/scholar_case?case=3952533722386911858&q=
David+S.+Tatum+v.+Takeda+Pharmaceuticals&hl=en&as_sdt=6,47

11. Becoming a Whistleblower

1. **Author**
Aaron S. Kesselheim
Year published:
2010
Article title:
Whistle-Blowers' Experiences in Fraud Litigation against Pharmaceutical Companies
Journal title:
New England Journal of Medicine
Issue number:
19
Volume number:
362
Pages:
1832-1839
2. **Author**
Angela Duckworth
Year published:
2017
Book title:
Grit
City:
[Place of publication not identified]
Publisher:
Vermilion
3. **Author**
Stephen M Kohn
Year published:
n.d.
Book title:

The new whistleblower's handbook

12. History of the False Claims Act

1. **Author**
   Stephen M Kohn
   Year published:
   n.d.
   Book title:
   The new whistleblower's handbook
2. **Author**
   Stephen M Kohn
   Year published:
   n.d.
   Book title:
   The new whistleblower's handbook
3. https://www.congress.gov/bill/114th-congress/senate-resolution/522/text
4. **Author**
   Stephen M Kohn
   Year published:
   n.d.
   Book title:
   The new whistleblower's handbook
5. **Author**
   John T Boese
   Year published:
   2000
   Book title:
   Civil false claims and qui tam actions
   City:
   Gaithersburg
   Publisher:
   Aspen Law & Business
6. **Author**
   Stephen M Kohn
   Year published:
   n.d.
   Book title:
   The new whistleblower's handbook
7. **Author**
   Stephen M Kohn
   Year published:
   n.d.

Book title:
The new whistleblower's handbook
8. **Author**
Stephen M Kohn
Year published:
n.d.
Book title:
The new whistleblower's handbook
9. **Author**
Stephen M Kohn
Year published:
n.d.
Book title:
The new whistleblower's handbook
10. https://scholar.google.com/scholar_case?case=10313675310414644402&q=
Allison+Engine+Co.+v.+United+States+ex+rel.+Sanders&hl=en&
as_sdt=20000006
11. 5 J. Bus. & Tech. L. 125 (2010)
Saying What They Mean: The False Claims Act Amendments in the
Wake of Allison Engine
https://heinonline.org/HOL/LandingPage?handle=hein.journals/
jobtela5&div=12&id=&page=
12. gladwell, m. (2018). [Podcast].
13. **Author**
Frederick L Hoffman
Year published:
1918
Book title:
Mortality from respiratory diseases in dusty trades
14. https://www.thefcainsider.com/2015/04/6-key-considerations-relating-to-
government-intervention-in-false-claims-cases/
15. https://www.americanbar.org/groups/litigation/committees/health-law/
articles/2014/winter2015-the-growing-threat-of-qui-tam-litigation-against-
healthcare-providers/

13. Rheumatologists

1. https://www.rheumatology.org/
2. **Author**
C.J. Hawkey
Year published:
2001
Article title:

COX-1 and COX-2 inhibitors
Journal title:
Best Practice & Research Clinical Gastroenterology
Issue number:
5
Volume number:
15
Pages:
801-820

3. **Author**

John Abramson
Year published:
2014
Book title:
Overdosed america
City:
[Place of publication not identified]
Publisher:
Harper Perennial

4. **Author**

Fred E. Silverstein
Year published:
2000
Article title:
Gastrointestinal Toxicity With Celecoxib vs Nonsteroidal Anti-inflammatory Drugs for Osteoarthritis and Rheumatoid Arthritis
Journal title:
JAMA
Issue number:
10
Volume number:
284
Pages:
1247

5. **Author**

Claire Bombardier
Year published:
2000
Article title:
Comparison of Upper Gastrointestinal Toxicity of Rofecoxib and Naproxen in Patients with Rheumatoid Arthritis
Journal title:
New England Journal of Medicine
Issue number:

21

Volume number:

343

Pages:

1520-1528

6. **Author**

R.S. Bresalier

Year published:

2005

Article title:

Cardiovascular Events Associated With Rofecoxib in a Colorectal Adenoma Chemoprevention Trial

Journal title:

ACC Current Journal Review

Issue number:

6

Volume number:

14

Pages:

5

7. https://www.mdedge.com/rheumatologynews/article/164177/rheumatoid-arthritis/fda-advisory-committee-votes-recommend-update

16. The Eastern District of Virginia

1. https://votesmart.org/public-statement/366197/senators-warner-and-webb-welcome-nomination-of-anthony-trenga-to-the-eastern-district-court-of-virginia#.W_W39ZM3nOQ

2. **Author**

Jeremy Gersh

Article title:

Saying What They Mean: The False Claims Act Amendments in the Wake of Allison Engine

Website title:

DigitalCommons@UM Carey Law

URL:

https://digitalcommons.law.umaryland.edu/jbtl/vol5/iss1/9/

19. The Solicitor General of the United States

1. http://www.scotusblog.com/2012/05/scotus-for-law-students-what-does-the-solicitor-general-do-sponsored-by-bloomberg-law/

2. http://www.scotusblog.com/2012/05/scotus-for-law-students-what-does-the-solicitor-general-do-sponsored-by-bloomberg-law/
3. http://www.scotusblog.com/2012/05/scotus-for-law-students-what-does-the-solicitor-general-do-sponsored-by-bloomberg-law/

21. Cases referring to Nathan v. Takeda

1. https://www.healthlawyers.org/find-a-resource/HealthLawHub/Documents/Compliance/FHL_paulhus.docx
2. https://www.leagle.com/decision/infdco20180427a77
3. https://scholar.google.com/scholar_case?case=13480565013166810771&q=United+States+Ex+Rel.+Ryan+v.+Endo+Pharma.&hl=en&as_sdt=20000003
4. https://scholar.google.com/scholar_case?case=13480565013166810771&q=United+States+Ex+Rel.+Ryan+v.+Endo+Pharma.&hl=en&as_sdt=20000003
5. https://scholar.google.com/scholar_case?case=12075525434817279116&q=U.S.+ex+rel.+Palmieri+et+al+v.+Alpharma+Inc&hl=en&as_sdt=20000003
6. https://scholar.google.com/scholar_case?case=12075525434817279116&q=U.S.+ex+rel.+Palmieri+et+al+v.+Alpharma+Inc&hl=en&as_sdt=20000003
7. https://www.healthlawyers.org/find-a-resource/HealthLawHub/Documents/Compliance/FHL_paulhus.docx
8. https://www.leagle.com/decision/infdco20180427a77
9. https://scholar.google.com/scholar_case?case=13480565013166810771&q=United+States+Ex+Rel.+Ryan+v.+Endo+Pharma.&hl=en&as_sdt=20000003
10. https://scholar.google.com/scholar_case?case=12075525434817279116&q=U.S.+ex+rel.+Palmieri+et+al+v.+Alpharma+Inc&hl=en&as_sdt=20000003

22. Articles referring to Nathan v. Takeda

1. **Author**
   Stephen M Kohn
   Year published:
   n.d.
   Book title:
   The new whistleblower's handbook
2. Particularity Discovery in Qui Tam Actions: A Middle Ground Approach to Pleading Fraud in the Health Care Sector - PennLawReview.com
   Website title:
   Pennlawreview.com
   URL:
   https://www.pennlawreview.com/print/?id=569
3. **Article title:**
   Particularity Discovery in Qui Tam Actions: A Middle Ground

Approach to Pleading Fraud in the Health Care Sector - PennLawReview.com
   Website title:
   Pennlawreview.com
   URL:
   https://www.pennlawreview.com/print/?id=569
4. https://www.healthlawyers.org/find-a-resource/HealthLawHub/
   Documents/Compliance/FHL_paulhus.docx
5. https://www.healthlawyers.org/find-a-resource/HealthLawHub/
   Documents/Compliance/FHL_paulhus.docx
6. **Author**
   Supreme Claims
   Article title:
   Supreme Court Declines to Opine on Circuit Split Over Rule 9(b)
   Pleading Requirements for FCA Claims
   Website title:
   Epstein Becker & Green
   URL:
   https://www.ebglaw.com/news/supreme-court-declines-to-opine-on-
   circuit-split-over-rule-9b-pleading-requirements-for-fca-claims/
7. **Author**
   Supreme Claims
   Article title:
   Supreme Court Declines to Opine on Circuit Split Over Rule 9(b)
   Pleading Requirements for FCA Claims
   Website title:
   Epstein Becker & Green
   URL:
   https://www.ebglaw.com/news/supreme-court-declines-to-opine-on-
   circuit-split-over-rule-9b-pleading-requirements-for-fca-claims/
8. **Website title:**
   Americanbar.org
   URL:
   https://www.americanbar.org/content/dam/aba/administrative/
   public_contract_law/
   2013_fall_meeting_leadership_portal/06_berger_BNA_article_pending_FCA
   _petitions.pdf
9. **Website title:**
   Americanbar.org
   URL:
   https://www.americanbar.org/content/dam/aba/administrative/
   public_contract_law/
   2013_fall_meeting_leadership_portal/06_berger_BNA_article_pending_FCA
   _petitions.pdf

10. https://scholarlycommons.law.northwestern.edu/cgi/viewcontent.cgi?
   article=1007&context=nulr

11. https://scholarlycommons.law.northwestern.edu/cgi/viewcontent.cgi?
   article=1007&context=nulr

12. **Article title:**
   In Defense of a Strict Pleading Standard for False Claims Act Whistle-
   blowers | The University of Chicago Law Review
   Website title:
   Lawreview.uchicago.edu
   URL:
   https://lawreview.uchicago.edu/publication/defense-strict-pleading-
   standard-false-claims-act-whistleblowers-4

13. **Article title:**
   In Defense of a Strict Pleading Standard for False Claims Act Whistle-
   blowers | The University of Chicago Law Review
   Website title:
   Lawreview.uchicago.edu
   URL:
   https://lawreview.uchicago.edu/publication/defense-strict-pleading-
   standard-false-claims-act-whistleblowers-4

14. https://heinonline.org/HOL/LandingPage?handle=hein.journals/
   geojlap13&div=2&id=&page=

15. https://heinonline.org/HOL/LandingPage?handle=hein.journals/
   geojlap13&div=2&id=&page=

16. **Article title:**
   Third Circuit Adds to Circuit Split on Rule 9(b)'s Particularity Require-
   ment in the Context of an FCA Claim | Meaningful Discussions
   Website title:
   Meaningful Discussions
   URL:
   https://www.meaningfuldiscussions.com/third-circuit-adds-to-circuit-
   split-on-rule-9bs-particularity-requirement-in-the-context-of-an-fca-claim/

17. **Article title:**
   Third Circuit Adds to Circuit Split on Rule 9(b)'s Particularity Require-
   ment in the Context of an FCA Claim | Meaningful Discussions
   Website title:
   Meaningful Discussions
   URL:
   https://www.meaningfuldiscussions.com/third-circuit-adds-to-circuit-
   split-on-rule-9bs-particularity-requirement-in-the-context-of-an-fca-claim/

23. Lupron

1. **Author**
   Elisabeth Rosenthal
   Year published:
   2017
   Book title:
   An American sickness
2. **Author**
   Elisabeth Rosenthal
   Year published:
   2017
   Book title:
   An American sickness
3. https://abcnews.go.com/WNT/story?id=130940&page=1

24. Actos (pioglitazone)

1. https://law.justia.com/cases/federal/district-courts/louisiana/lawdce/6:
   2012cv00064/121414/686/
2. https://www.fda.gov/Drugs/DrugSafety/ucm259150.htm

25. Conclusion - Call To Action

1. https://scholar.google.com/scholar_case?case=10313675310414644402&q=
   Allison+Engine+Co.+v.+United+States+ex+rel.+Sanders&hl=en&
   as_sdt=20000006
2. 5 J. Bus. & Tech. L. 125 (2010)
   Saying What They Mean: The False Claims Act Amendments in the
   Wake of Allison Engine
   https://heinonline.org/HOL/LandingPage?handle=hein.journals/
   jobtela5&div=12&id=&page=

ACKNOWLEDGMENTS

Needless to say, this entire process wouldn't have happened if I didn't have attorneys in my life. With the incredible stress of the situation, it is not uncommon for people in this scenario to have major life-changing events. I was married to an attorney for almost fourteen years, and we have two amazing boys who are now teenagers. If I didn't have her in my life at the time, this adventure would have never taken place, Thank you! While at Georgetown Law School she was close friends with two other law students that would eventually get married, Jennifer and James Bell.

We became very good friends with Jen & Jim and would vacation together. They eventually started their own firm in Philadelphia, PA, Bell & Bell LLP.

Bell & Bell LLP was our partner with the whole process. It was costly to bring the case to trial with needing local counsel, expert witnesses, *qui tam* research, *qui tam* appellate attorneys, deposition costs, travel costs, etc... not even accounting for the incredible number of their legal hours.

In the process of writing this book, I asked Jim if he would do it again? He thought about it and said "yes." It was the right thing to do.

I also need to thank our appellate legal team of MoloLamken LLP from Washington, DC. Jeffrey Lamken took the lead with Michael Pattillo, Jr as his second chair. They did an incredible job bringing the case through the 4th Circuit Court of Appeals as well as writing the Cert-Petition to the United States Supreme Court. The Supreme Court was interested in taking my case and sent it to the Solicitor General of the United States for his feedback. Unfortunately, the Court declined to take my case but I can't fault my team.

I want to thank John Drake from J Drake Graphic Design (https://jdrakegraphicdesign.com) in Richmond, VA. John is a fraternity brother of mine that I reached out to for help in designing a cover for the book, and he came up with a great one. I picture the pills coming out of the whistle as notes coming out of a song bird.

The case started in 2009 and ended in 2014. I am writing this book in 2018 and have a new outlook on life. After so many years of hiding the fact that I was a whistleblower, I am now embracing it. I tried to do the right thing which is what we should all strive for. I am currently engaged to my Best Friend and couldn't be happier. I want to thank Shara Alpert for her love and support while I wrote this book and look forward to our future together.